Advanced Life Support Skills

Advanced Life Support Skills

Editor

E. Jackson Allison, Jr., MD/MPH, FACEP

Sterling Distinguished Professor & Chair
Department of Emergency Medicine
East Carolina University School of Medicine
Chief of Service
Emergency Department
Pitt County Memorial Hospital
Greenville, North Carolina
Past President of
American College of
Emergency Physicians

Authors

Dwight A. Polk, BA, NREMT-P

Paramedic Program Coordinator
Department of Emergency Health Services
University of Maryland Baltimore County
Baltimore, Maryland

Mary Gardner, RN, MICN, EMT-P

ALS Coordinator
Division of Emergency Medical Services
Department of Emergency Medical Services
East Carolina University School of Medicine
Greenville, North Carolina

Richard C. Hunt, MD, FACEP

Assistant Professor and Chief
Division of Air Medical Services
Department of Emergency Medicine
East Carolina University School of Medicine
Greenville, North Carolina

N. Heramba Prasad, MD, FACEP

Medical Director
Division of Emergency Medical Services
Department of Emergency Medical Services
East Carolina University School of Medicine
Greenville, North Carolina

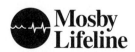
Mosby Lifeline

St. Louis Baltimore Boston Chicago London Madrid Philadelphia Sydney Toronto

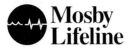
**Mosby
Lifeline**

Dedicated to Publishing Excellence

Publisher: David T. Culverwell
Editor: Claire Merrick
Developmental Editor: Nancy Peterson
Assistant Editor: Dana Battaglia
Project Manager: Gayle May Morris
Production Editor: Mary Cusick Drone
Manufacturing Supervisor: Betty Richmond
Designer: Susan Lane

Cover Photo: Thomas Cooper/*Emergency*

Printed in the United States of America
Composition by The Clarinda Company
Printing/binding by Maple Vail—Binghamton

Mosby—Year Book, Inc.
11830 Westline Industrial Drive
St. Louis, Missouri 63146

Library of Congress Cataloging-in-Publication Data

Advanced life support skills / chief editor, E. Jackson Allison, Jr. ;
    editors, Dwight A. Polk . . . [et al.].
        p.   cm.
    Includes bibliographical references and index.
    ISBN 0-8016-7426-3
    1. Emergency medicine.   2. Emergency medical technicians.
    I. Allison, E. Jackson.
        [DNLM: 1. Emergencies.   2. Emergency Medical Services—methods.
    WB 105 A244   1994]
    RC86.7.A34   1994
    616.02'5—dc20
    DNLM/DLC
    for Library of Congress   93-19346
                                                                              CIP

94 95 96 97 98   9 8 7 6 5 4 3 2

To Sue Wilson, whose life support, both basic and advanced,
has resuscitated me occasionally and sustained me indefinitely through all
times,
good and bad, great and small.
E.J.A.

To my mother, Jeanette, to the memory of my father, John,
and to the world's greatest support system:
Simon, Nick, Patti, Patrick, John, Maggie, Joe, and Wayne,
who were always there with a word of encouragement when I needed to hear a
stable voice. And to my students, who constantly remind me why I still love this
crazy profession after 19 years!
D.A.P.

To my parents, Paul and Fran Ludowese,
for always supporting me and encouraging me to reach for the stars.
To Michelle and Lisa, my "EMS Children"
who have always been a source of love and support. To all my students
who have challenged me and taught me something new in every class.
M.G.

To my friends and mentors, Jack and Nick, who have shown me the way.
To my parents, whose faith in me makes me persevere.
To my wife, Gail, who sheds new light on my work,
and continually reinforces its value and whose love is constant.
To my son, Wes, whose insights even in adolescence
stimulate me to be more creative.
To my daughter, Emily, who makes me smile and laugh,
and who reminds me of why we're here.
R.C.H.

To my wife Barbara, who endures enormous suffering on my behalf
and still finds ways to love me; and my children, Michael, Yasmine,
and Marissa. I love you all dearly.
N.H.P.

Foreword

Only a few years ago, if an individual experienced a health emergency outside the hospital, a heart attack or injuries in a motor vehicle crash, little if any medical care was provided before the ill or injured patient arrived at the hospital. This lack of prehospital emergency medical care resulted in many unnecessary deaths. Over the past two decades, the situation has changed dramatically for the better. Two major forces in the early 1970s led to unprecedented growth and development of emergency medical services (EMS) in this country. Federal funding provided many systems with the capital necessary to develop an EMS infrastructure. Simultaneously, the television show, *Emergency,* mesmerized the American public. Roy and Johnnie routinely demonstrated how properly trained health care providers could bring lifesaving skills and technology to the streets. They became national heroes and the envy of many impressionable viewers, ranging from children to city planners. Dollars and good intentions, however, were not enough to allow a rational and scientific development of this new medical specialty of prehospital care. Equipment was frequently chosen on the basis of salesmen, without regard for the knowledge and skill that make a medical device worthy. Roy and Johnnie had few EMS texts from which to choose. A wide variety of medical paraphernalia were pedalled without sound, scientific basis for use or proper educational materials to guarantee correct use. Medical protocols were frequently written as a hobby by well-meaning token physicians.

By its very nature, prehospital emergency medical care is "skill" oriented. Prehospital providers save lives and alleviate suffering because they have skills that allow them to secure and maintain an airway, treat life-threatening dysrhythmias, and gain vascular access. Prehospital skills have evolved to an exceedingly advanced level. As with any field using advanced skills, providers of prehospital EMS face the challenge of learning and maintaining the skills necessary to achieve the desired outcome. Skill acquisition and maintenance are critical in EMS since the desired outcomes, the prevention of unnecessary death and disability, and the relief of pain and suffering have utmost importance.

The level of prehospital care provided "in the streets" has advanced faster than the educational materials necessary for skill development and maintenance. Of all the textbooks available for prehospital educators and providers, there are few devoted exclusively to the area of EMS that probably has the greatest impact—advanced prehospital skills. Jack Allison, Sterling Distinguished Professor & Chair of Emergency Medicine at East Carolina University and a long-time EMS proponent, has put a text together to help fill that void. Considering the authors are all active members of the prehospital team (i.e., physicians, educators, and providers), there is little doubt that this text will have value both in the classroom and "in the streets."

The text has several unique features that add to its value. First and foremost are the more than 500 photographs and drawings that illustrate in a step-by-step fashion exactly how to perform advanced prehospital skills. Another unique and valuable feature is the "Pearls and Pitfalls" boxes included in each chapter that contain practical tips that really work—tips that usually come from years of experience in the field. The question and answer section for each chapter is another unique feature of this text that allows providers to test themselves.

As we approach the new millennium, pre-hospital care is continuing to evolve and mature. Fortunately, we are now enjoying the creation of quality resources such as *Advanced Life Support Skills*. This text provides the bricks from which to develop a strong educational foundation. Both students and seasoned providers will benefit from the breadth of information presented in a reader-friendly manner. The authors have done a remarkable job of combining reliable, state-of-the-art information with the streetwise perspective of seasoned clinicians. The skills and knowledge of EMS providers are the first and frequently the most important link in the chain of care. This text will go a long way toward strengthening all of the links in the emergency health care chain. EMS is finally growing from a field based on anecdote and intuition to one based on research and sound clinical doctrine.

Paul M. Paris, MD, FACEP

Associate Professor and Chief
Division of Emergency Medicine
University of Pittsburgh School of Medicine
Chief Medical Officer/Interim Chief Executive Officer
Center for Emergency Medicine of Western
  Pennsylvania
Immediate Past President, National Association of EMS
  Physicians
Medical Director, City of Pittsburgh
Department of Public Safety
Pittsburgh, Pennsylvania

Foreword

Two vital pieces of "equipment" provide the keys to success for a prehospital professional: a sharp mind and skillful hands. The professional's mind requires education, but the hands require careful and thorough training. For the technician to provide the lifesaving or stabilizing interventions that he knows must be provided, his hands must be ready to perform. Training in skill performance is a critical portion of their preparation.

Every member of the prehospital care team is keenly aware of the importance of advanced life support skills. Airway interventions are paramount in sustaining life and a viable brain. Intravenous access provides the means to replace lost vascular volume and administer necessary medications. Each skill described in this book requires careful judgment in its application to a particular patient and precision in its execution.

This text provides an exceptional training format for the prehospital professional's skills.

By dissecting each skill down to its essential core and offering an inventory of pearls and pitfalls, the authors guide their readers to competence in these skills. The emphasis is on everyday skills used routinely by technicians across this nation.

Using photographs and illustrations frequently though the manual brings the material to life and clarifies many of the mysteries of these procedures. Technicians from traditional ground EMS services, from air medical transport services, from urban providers, and from rural regions with extended transport times will all find this an exceptional teaching tool.

Nicholas H. Benson, MD, FACEP

Associate Professor and Vice Chair
Department of Emergency Medicine
East Carolina University School of Medicine;
Medical Director
North Carolina Office of Emergency Medical Services;
President Elect
National Association of Emergency Medical Services
   Physicians

Preface

When I was first invited by Mosby to edit this text, my initial reaction was one of unabashed excitement. Now, some four years later, I'm even more delighted about this, the first edition of this book, for there is indeed a palpable need on the street, and even in the Emergency Department for a practical, straightforward advanced life support (ALS) skills and equipment textbook.

I chose Dwight Polk, Mary Gardner, Rick Hunt, and Heramba Prasad as authors because they are experienced, knowledgeable, dedicated, and exemplary EMS educators and practitioners. The fact that they are excellent writers was also a plus!

This textbook is based on new concepts in EMS education, especially in the realm of teaching ALS skills and recommending basic equipment. The accompanying original photographs and illustrations were chosen to enhance the simplified, step-by-step approach to patient assessment and management primarily in the prehospital phase of emergency medical care. The fundamental goals are twofold: to help new ALS personnel become "street savvy," and to provide more seasoned providers with a quick update/refresher.

It's often been said that writing a book is comparable to giving birth: the process is long, uncertain, anxiety provoking, and rather painful—yet, over 95% of the time the final outcome is a joyous miracle. Personally I have been afforded an excellent team, including the four authors, as well as an absolutely superb staff at Mosby that made the process rewarding and successful.

We encourage you to read this book and enjoy it. It is our hope and belief that it will become dogeared very soon from frequent use, first as an illustrated how-to, hands-on baseline ALS textbook, and second as a subsequent quick reference text.

We're already looking forward to revising future editions. Cheers!!

E. Jackson Allison, Jr. MD/MPH, FACEP

Acknowledgments

*We are indebted to many people whose significant contributions
made this book possible.*

First and foremost, Kathleen A. Cline, MD, FACEP, provided expert consultation regarding ALS communications, patient assessment, and the approach to neonatal and pediatric patients. Her pearls of wisdom are so evident, and very much appreciated.

Dave Balch and the entire staff of the Center for Health Sciences Communications were invaluable in providing all of the artwork in the book. More specifically, Alan Branigan and Betty Mayers worked tirelessly on the illustrations, and John Artois was masterful in his medical photography. John is also blessed with the enviable virtues of patience and diligence!

Barry Bunn, EMT-P, is also a medical student at East Carolina University School of Medicine. Barry's contributions to this book were manifold: he wrote the drug calculation, radio report, and documentation sections; and he spent untold hours in helping us shoot the photos. Barry has always strived to make EMS clinically challenging, socially responsible, and intellectually stimulating.

We are most appreciative of the professional guidance and infinite patience of Mosby's senior editorial staff, including Claire Merrick, Nancy Peterson, Dana Battaglia, Mary Drone, and Susan Lane.

Finally, we could not have accomplished this book without the professional manuscript preparation by our talented secretarial staff: Kay Cyrus, Patricia Furman, Beth Denton and Kim Page.

Publisher's Acknowledgments

The editors wish to acknowledge the following reviewers of this book
for their invaluable help in developing and fine-tuning the manuscript.

Thomas P. Butcher, Jr., RN, MPH, NREMP-T
Clinical Nurse III
Emergency Department
Touro Infirmary
New Orleans, Louisiana
Guest Faculty
Elaine P. Nunez Technical Institute
Chalmette, Louisiana

Debra Cason, RN, MS, EMT-P
Associate Professor
Program Director
Emergency Medicine Education
University of Texas Southwestern Medical Center
Dallas, Texas

Robert Elling, MPA, NREMT-P
Senior EMS Representative
NYS EMS Program
Albany, New York

Kevin Kraus, BS, EMT-P
Associate Planner
New York State Emergency Management Office
Division of Military and Naval Affairs
Albany, New York

Baxter Larmon, MS, MICP
Assistant Professor of Medicine
Associate Director
UCLA Center for Prehospital Care
Los Angeles, California

Paul M. Maniscalco
D/C Commanding Officer
Special Operations Division
City of New York Emergency Medical Service
New York, New York

Keith Neely
Department of Emergency Services
Oregon Health Sciences University
Portland, Oregon

William D. Ramsey, MD, FACEP
Assistant Professor of Emergency Medicine
Department of Surgery
West Virginia University Health Sciences Center
Morgantown, West Virginia
Regional Medical Director Region VI-VII
West Virginia EMS System
Chairman of West Virginia State Curriculum and
Training Committee
West Virginia

William Raynovich, MPH, BS, Masters in Public
Health, NREMT-P
Director of Prehospital Services
The Reading Hospital and Medical Center
West Reading, Pennsylvania

Kevin H. Scruggs, MD
Emergency Medicine Department
Franklin Square Hospital Center
Baltimore, Maryland

Contents

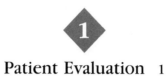
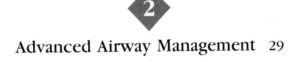

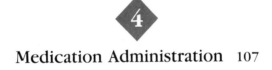
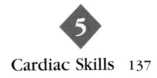
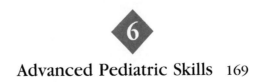

APPENDIXES

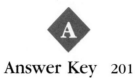

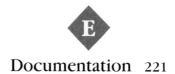

Documentation 221

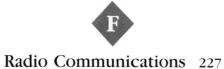

Radio Communications 227

National Registry of EMT/Paramedic Examination Skill Sheets 235

American Heart Association Advanced Life Support Algorithms 249

Advanced Life Support Skills

◆ A Note to the Reader

The authors and publisher have made every attempt to check dosages and advanced life support content for accuracy. The care procedures presented here represent accepted practices in the United States. They are not offered as a standard of care. Advanced life support level emergency care is performed under the authority of a licensed physician. It is the reader's responsibility to know and to follow local care protocols as provided by their medical advisers. It is also the reader's responsibility to stay informed of emergency care procedure changes.

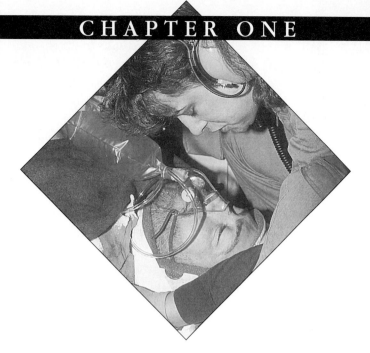

CHAPTER ONE

Patient Evaluation

Objectives

A paramedic should be able to—

1. Identify situations in which patient evaluation and management should be expedited.

2. List three similarities between patient evaluation and documentation techniques.

3. List six stages of patient evaluation.

4. List four safety tips that can be used at the scene to ensure the safety of EMS and supportive personnel.

5. Differentiate between the assessment techniques used for patients of medical and trauma emergencies.

6. Evaluate and manage a patient on the basis of the following steps: primary survey, primary resuscitation, secondary survey, secondary resuscitation.

7. List two reasons for patient reevaluation after initial treatment.

8. Differentiate between two styles of documentation.

Photo courtesy Don B. Stevenson/*Emergency.*

Case Scenario

Your unit is dispatched to an area just south of town to an automobile crash involving a bicycle. Dispatch advises you that the patient is not moving, according to sources at the scene.

On approaching the crash site, you can see a small child lying next to a bicycle. As you approach the patient, you note that a young male, approximately 6 years old, is motionless and cyanotic. His breathing is noisy and stridorous. You tell the patient to lie still as you stabilize his head and cervical spine, but he doesn't seem to respond to your voice or touch. You manage his airway by manually opening it with a modified jaw-thrust to clear the stridor. You immediately suction the oropharynx, insert an oropharyngeal airway, and apply oxygen at 15 L/minute via a nonrebreather mask. His respiratory status improves, and breathing becomes easier. You expose the chest and note that the chest rises on the left, but not the right. You examine the back using a modified logroll. You find a puncture wound on the right side near the eighth rib and a large contusion over the right flank. You seal the open wound with a defibrillator pad and bulky dressing, and logroll him back to the supine position. Breath sounds are present bilaterally, but they are still slightly decreased on the right side. Color has not improved; thus you intubate the patient and ventilate him with a bag-valve mask (BVM) and 100% oxygen.

His carotid pulses are rapid and thready, and his radials are absent. Capillary refill time is 3 seconds. The skin is cold and clammy. You rapidly examine him from head-to-toe for other gross signs of injury and find none. He still does not respond to your voice and only groans with sternal rub.

You decide to rapidly package and transport the patient to a trauma center. A cervical collar is placed, a pediatric pneumatic antishock garment (PASG) is applied with only the legs inflated, and the patient is secured to a spine board. En route to the hospital, you obtain vital signs. Pulse oximetry shows an SaO$_2$ of 90, blood pressure (BP) is 60/42, respirations are assisted, and EKG shows sinus tachycardia.

You complete the secondary survey, finding no additional injuries. Following protocol, you initiate bilateral intravenous lines (IVs) of lactated Ringer's and continue ventilatory assistance. Respiratory compliance and vital signs are monitored closely in anticipation of a developing tension pneumothorax.

You arrive at the trauma center with no further deterioration in condition. Rapid evaluation by the receiving physician affirms the field evaluation and treatment. A chest tube is inserted into the patient's right midaxillary chest wall at the fourth intercostal space, resulting in immediate improvement in respirations. Diagnostic laboratory work and x-rays are obtained. Whole blood is given, and the patient is taken to surgery within 10 minutes of arrival. After a few weeks of recuperation, he is allowed to return to school on a regular basis.

Patient evaluation is one skill that an advanced prehospital care provider will use on every emergency response. Yet it is a skill that often is performed incompletely or haphazardly. Without a thorough understanding of patient evaluation, the remaining skills in this book would be useless. Assessment is the cornerstone of all patient care.

This chapter emphasizes the importance of a thorough and consistent patient evaluation, while allowing for variations according to the specific situation at hand. Advanced care entails much more than the dexterity of performing advanced skills; the insight and judgment that help decide when to apply these skills are also critically important.

◆ Stages of Patient Evaluation

The concept of evaluation in the prehospital setting goes beyond that of simply determining what is wrong with the patient. To provide total care, a paramedic should accomplish six stages of patient evaluation by the completion of the emergency run. These six stages are:

- Evaluation of the scene

- Identification of life-threatening illness or injury
- Rapid intervention
- Comprehensive assessment
- Treatment and transportation
- Reevaluation

Generally speaking, the first three stages are performed in the order listed. The latter three may occur at various times throughout the call or simultaneously, depending on the situation. It should be noted, however, that in special cases, such as an auto crash near a hospital, all six stages may not be accomplished. There is no justification, especially in trauma, for remaining at the scene for an excessive period of time to fulfill all six stages when an emergency department is only 5 minutes away.

Stage 1: Evaluation of the Scene

Before any direct patient contact, crew members should be alert for potential hazards to responding personnel and the patient. Hazards such as emotionally charged family members, unstable vehicles, or hazardous chemical conditions must be dealt with before placing crew personnel in jeopardy. Additional Emergency Medical Services (EMSs) and fire units, hazardous materials teams, and utility companies should be called for assistance if necessary. Rescuer safety should always be kept in the forefront of any emergency response. An injured responder can tax the resources of an EMS system, since extra units will be required to treat and transport both you and the original patient.

At the scene of an emergency response, observation is one of the most important tools for a paramedic to use. Important information about injuries or medical conditions can be obtained simply by surveying the environment. The observant paramedic should be attuned to unusual odors, sights, and sounds. For example, items such as empty medicine bottles or insulin syringes can provide much needed information about the unresponsive diabetic patient who has no family present. Similarly, noting

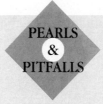

Scene Safety

There are many safety tips that can be used at the scene to prevent a paramedic from becoming a victim. Here are a few:

- Assess hazards of the scene before charging in!
- Never knock on a door while standing directly in front of it—always stand to the side.
- Never approach a night scene with a flashlight directly in front of you...always hold it out to your side to prevent making yourself a direct target.
- Always have someone lead you to the patient. Never become the victim for an upset patient who is waiting in a dark room.
- When a patient is in a vehicle (other than when you are responding to an auto crash), make an effort to write down the license plate number before departing the unit.
- Beware of animals. The most gentle of pets will often bite if it thinks its owner is being threatened. Have it removed by family members.
- Always park your unit at an angle that will allow for rapid departure in case the scene rapidly deteriorates.
- Never be in a position that has your back toward an open door—always keep your back to a wall.
- Do not let the patient get between you and the door.
- Be aware that tools of the trade such as scissors, folding knives, and stethoscopes can be used as weapons by a hostile patient.

odors such as those from a kerosene heater or automobile exhaust fumes may suggest carbon monoxide poisoning. Whenever two or more crew members have simultaneous symptoms, it strongly suggests an environmental gas or agent. Crews should always report any symptoms to fellow crew members immediately. Delays can be **DEADLY!**

Stages 2 and 3: Identification of Life-Threatening Illness/Injury and Rapid Intervention

After securing the scene, the next two steps in patient evaluation often occur simultaneously. The paramedic must rapidly identify any life-threatening illnesses or injuries that the patient may have incurred. This procedure is commonly termed the primary survey. If signs and symptoms of a serious illness or injury are recognized, immediate action is required. This action is the primary resuscitation. Only those illnesses and injuries that pose a life-threatening condition should receive treatment at this point; less serious conditions are identified and managed later in the call.

The primary survey can be seen as a step-by-step "global" overview of the patient's respiratory, circulatory, and neurologic status. The paramedic should begin with a 15-second rapid survey to understand the situation and the general condition of the patient. This is accomplished by a quick assessment of the respiratory pattern of the patient, the presence of carotid and radial pulses, the presence of any major hemorrhage, and the patient's response to a paramedic (Figure 1-1).

The actual primary survey occurs next and is based on five distinct steps:
1. Airway control (and cervical spine control, if needed)
2. Breathing
3. Circulation and hemorrhage control
4. Disability (mini-neurologic examination)
5. Exposure and examination

It is important for a paramedic to identify himself or herself when approaching any patient. Communication between the prehospital care provider and the patient should never cease from that point. Research has shown that many senses—especially hearing—continue

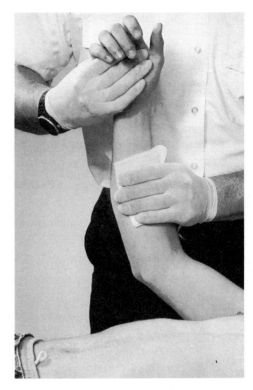

Figure 1-1 Evaluating the circulatory system and controlling major hemorrhage are accomplished in the primary phase of patient evaluation.

to function even in patients who appear to be unresponsive. Try to elicit a response from every patient. Striking up a conversation with the responsive patient can give valuable information, as can shaking and shouting at the unresponsive patient.

The patient's *airway* must then be addressed, and every effort must be made to ensure that it is secure and patent. This step may also require cervical spine stabilization if the patient is suspected of having sustained spinal trauma (Figure 1-2, *A*). For example, a patient who has a stroke and falls down a flight of stairs meets these criteria, even though the foremost problem is medical. The use of the modified jaw-thrust or chin-lift maneuver is appropriate in an unresponsive patient and may be the only procedure needed to establish patency. In the event of obvious facial trauma or the presence of mucus or emesis, immediate suctioning is in-

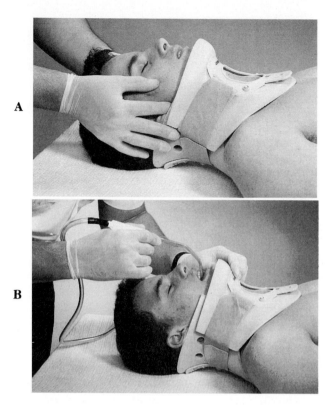

Figure 1-2 A, Use the modified jaw thrust to maintain the airway in patients with suspected cervical trauma. **B,** Suctioning with a rigid-tip catheter.

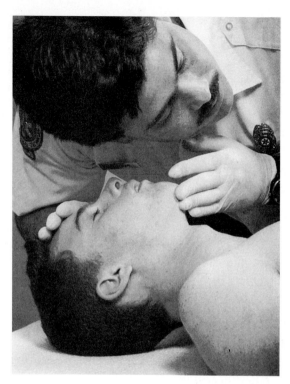

Figure 1-3 Open the airway—look, listen, and feel for air exchange.

dicated (Figure 1-2, *B*). However, a person talking normally can be assumed to have a patent airway and no life-threatening chest injury.

The evaluation of a patient's *breathing* capability is performed by looking, listening, and feeling. In doing so, it is important to determine not only if the patient is moving air, but if the effort is adequate (Figure 1-3).

To begin, listen. Noisy breathing indicates airway compromise. Audible sounds, such as stridor or wheezing, can suggest upper airway obstruction or asthma, respectively. Then expose the chest and look for movements or injuries that stand out, such as paradoxic movement or open injury sites. Contusions, flail segments, and tracheal deviation are key respiratory characteristics requiring immediate intervention. Anterior and posterior palpation of the chest wall for signs of loss of rib cage continuity is extremely important and can help identify a flail segment.

Confirmation of respiratory compromise can be accomplished by auscultating the chest and evaluating breath sounds. Is there air movement? What is its quality? Can you identify any extraordinary sounds? Absence of breath sounds in the thoracic cavity, accompanied by tracheal deviation, distended neck veins, and hyperresonance, suggests a tension pneumothorax. Similarly, a decrease in breath sounds accompanied by hyporesonance is indicative of a hemothorax.

In addition, the rate and depth of respirations should be assessed. Determination of successful air movement provides a paramedic with the necessary information to select the oxygen treatment modality for a patient. Before moving on to the next step in patient evaluation, the appropriate airway management therapy must be initiated. This includes insertion of an oropharyngeal airway, oxygen ad-

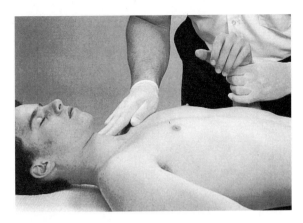

Figure 1-4 Simultaneously palpate a carotid and a radial pulse.

ministration, endotracheal intubation, needle cricothyrotomy, or chest decompression, as deemed necessary.

Circulatory assessment is the next step in patient evaluation. In performing the assessment, the respiratory and circulatory systems absolutely cannot be separated, since they are so interdependent. For example, evaluation of a patient's color not only determines whether cyanosis is present as a result of possible hypoxia, but it also can reveal a sign of poor hemoglobin status within the circulatory system.

The assessment of a patient's circulation encompasses several components: evaluation of the radial and carotid pulses, evaluation of peripheral perfusion, search for and treatment of major hemorrhage, initiation of fluid replacement, and PASG, if appropriate.

A comparison of the carotid and radial pulses provides a rapid initial assessment for early signs of shock (Figure 1-4). First, the presence or absence of both pulses is noted. When a carotid pulse is palpated, the patient has a systolic blood pressure of at least 60 mm Hg. Similarly, the presence of a radial pulse indicates a systolic reading of at least 80 mm Hg. Rate and quality of the pulses are then evaluated, not by specifically counting a rate, but by determin-

ing if the speed is bradycardic (<60) or tachycardic (>100). A thready or bounding pulse gives additional pertinent information about the circulatory condition.

At the same time, a paramedic can easily examine the patient's skin condition. Factors such as temperature, moisture, and capillary refill greater than 2 seconds are key indicators for shock. Hence, in a matter of seconds, it can be determined that a patient who has cool, clammy skin; 3-second capillary refill; weak, rapid carotid pulse; and absent radial pulse is in decompensated shock. The patient should be surveyed for external hemorrhage, and major bleeding should be controlled when identified.

The *primary resuscitation* phase begins again once shock is identified. Because shock is a major life-threatening situation that requires rapid intervention, PASG should be applied, provided the patient's respiratory status is not compromised or other contraindications do not exist. Further circulatory support should include the initiation of rapidly infused intravenous crystalloids (lactated Ringer's or normal saline), using the largest intravenous catheter possible. IVs should be initiated while en route to the hospital.

The *disability* step of the primary survey is generally accomplished by this point, simply by talking and working with the patient. This step serves as a mini-neurologic examination to further assess the patient's level of responsiveness. This is done by noting the patient's response to your presence and performing several simple evaluative procedures. The letters *A-V-P-U* are useful in assessing the patient's level of consciousness.

A = *A*lert
V = Responds to *v*erbal stimuli
P = Responds to *p*ainful stimuli
U = *U*nresponsive

To evaluate a patient's responsiveness, a paramedic needs to ask questions dealing with *persons, places,* and *things* that can be easily verified. Identification of family members or pets and their location is often a good method of assessment. A failure to recollect the date and time of day is a poor indicator for disorientation, since many people are unaware of time for various reasons. However, the questions may be asked, and a correct response is a positive sign of orientation.

A person is considered to respond appropriately to verbal stimuli when he or she responds to your verbal requests. Asking a patient to blink his eyes, or stick out his tongue is an excellent test that also serves to partially evaluate the cranial nerves.

Painful response implies that the patient has an intact central nervous system that responds to noxious or painful stimuli. Simple techniques such as pinching the nailbed or stroking the bottom of the foot may provide enough stimulus to elicit a response. Occasionally a paramedic may have to pinch the muscle just above the clavicle or perform a sternal rub to elicit a response (Figure 1-5, *A* and *B*).

Unresponsiveness is also determined on the basis of the same simple neurologic examination. A patient can then be classified as totally responsive, responsive to verbal and/or painful stimuli, or totally unresponsive. Evaluating level of consciousness (LOC) is extremely important for two reasons: (1) restlessness, anxiety, or agitation is usually one of the first signs to change with head injury or impending

Local Protocols

In the context of reading a skills manual, you must be aware that local or state protocols must be followed.

Cool skin temperature, cyanosis, and the absence of a carotid pulse indicate that your patient is in complete cardiopulmonary arrest. Your local or state protocol dictates whether cardiopulmonary resuscitation (CPR) should be initiated at this time or not, and what advanced life support (ALS) measures should be initiated.

Local or state protocols dictate under what conditions a paramedic may stop CPR. Decisions such as these are more complicated for the ALS provider than for basic providers. Some EMS systems allow the prehospital provider to terminate CPR if the complete arrest has been run through medical control. Others require that all patients be transported to the hospital. Each situation must be handled according to your system's protocol, but remember that each situation is different.

"Do not resuscitate," or DNR, orders are another area of concern for all providers. Each state should have detailed laws regarding this situation. Generally speaking, the prehospital provider is obligated to honor DNR requests, providing a family member or nurse has a written order. Oral DNR orders can only be honored in special circumstances by speaking directly to the family or receiving physician.

The PASG is another area of controversy in the prehospital arena. The argument continues about how successful it is in reversing shock. At the current time, the U. S. Department of Transportation (DOT) EMT-Paramedic: National Standard Curriculum recommends the use of the garment in obvious cases of shock. However, realize that your local or state protocol supersedes the DOT curriculum, since it is only a guideline.

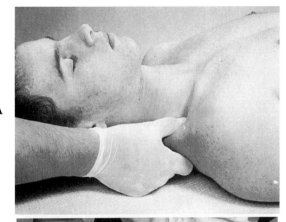

A

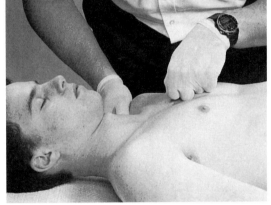

B

Figure 1-5 A, Pinch the area superior to the clavicle. **B,** Perform a sternal rub to gain a painful response.

shock; and (2) determining LOC gives the paramedic a baseline status with which to reevaluate the patient during treatment.

Exposure and examination are the final steps of the primary survey. These steps are often performed simultaneously with the evaluation of breathing and circulation. For example, on recognition of life-threatening illness or injury, many paramedics prefer that the patient's clothing be completely removed. This allows for prompt examination and treatment of critical sites. Global exposure and examination also serve as a fail-safe measure in case an injury was overlooked earlier in the survey. Any necessary exposure and examination can be performed at this time before continuing on to the comprehensive assessment. Every effort

PEARLS
&
PITFALLS

Excessive Stimulation

At no time should a paramedic go to extreme measures, such as pinching the skin with hemostats or applying excessive ammonia inhalant to elicit a response. Even if there is reason to believe that the patient is intentionally not responding to you, actions such as these are unethical and unprofessional.

should be made to preserve the patient's privacy and body heat.

Stage 4: Comprehensive Assessment

The purpose of the *comprehensive,* or *secondary, assessment* is to enable a paramedic to perform a detailed head-to-toe survey of the emergency patient. The comprehensive assessment can be modified according to the evaluation style of the paramedic, as well as the nature of the emergency. Systemic evaluations differ greatly between medical and trauma patients. For example, a patient complaining of substernal chest pain must be interviewed and assessed on the basis of probable cardiac problems. However, a patient who hit his chest on the steering wheel during an auto crash and complains of pain should be evaluated for possible thoracic injuries as well.

The physical examination process is based on four distinct skills: *inspection, auscultation, palpation,* and *percussion.* Each skill enables a paramedic to collect specific information that will assist in determining the probable cause of illness or injury.

Inspection is the visual examination. It should be performed first, since it is the most rapid and least invasive to accomplish and requires no special devices. A paramedic should

The Primary Survey

Paramedics must realize that in special cases they may never exit the primary phase.

For example, in cases of cardiac or traumatic arrest, the primary survey and primary resuscitation are initiated, and the patient is immobilized on a long spineboard and transported expeditiously to the most appropriate hospital. Time does not permit for detailed secondary surveys, prolonged history-taking, and minor treatments.

look for anything that is "abnormal" about the patient such as edema, bruises, deformities, and jaundice, as well as the normal findings.

Auscultation is the process of listening to sounds produced by the body and typically refers to the skill performed using the stethoscope. Since not all sounds are audible by the ear, a stethoscope is used to amplify the sound made by a specific organ. Even though many organs can be evaluated, auscultation of the lungs provides a paramedic with the most useful information. In a matter of seconds, the presence of rales, rhonchi, or wheezes can be made. By contrast, it often takes 5 to 10 minutes to perform a complete abdominal auscultatory evaluation.

Palpation uses the sense of touch and pressure to gather information about the patient. By using gentle technique, palpation allows the identification of tender areas, deformities, distention, and temperature. This "laying on of hands" is in many ways therapeutic and is an excellent way to gain patient trust.

Percussion involves tapping an object or area to invoke a vibration and subsequent sound waves. Percussion is not commonly used

in the field, since it requires a relatively quiet surrounding. However, if used, percussion is most beneficial in the evaluation of the chest in cases of suspected tension pneumothorax. Hyperresonance is heard as a result of the buildup of trapped air in the chest cavity. If hyporesonance is noted, it suggests the presence of blood in the pleural space, such as that found with a hemothorax.

The comprehensive assessment is made on the basis of information found in the primary survey. The secondary evaluation should be performed using a systematic, head-to-toe technique unless obvious injury or illness dictates care. A toe-to-head technique is often used with children. Every paramedic has his own preference for the most appropriate order in which to conduct a survey. In actuality, the patient's condition and surroundings should direct the evaluation, hence making every assessment different. To simplify the process, specific injuries and treatment modalities are discussed in later chapters.

Head and face

The head and cervical spine should be stabilized to prevent any spinal cord damage that could occur during the examination. The head and face should be inspected for any signs of deformity and bleeding by using a gloved hand to palpate the entire cranial and facial area (Figures 1-6 and 1-7). Special attention should be given to each of the sensory organs. The ears should be visualized for blood or cerebrospinal fluid, which is indicative of a possible basilar skull fracture. The eyes should be evaluated for pupillary size and response, as well as for accommodation (Figure 1-8). The nose should be inspected for symmetry and any signs of blood, mucus, or cerebrospinal fluid that could create airway problems. If found, the airway should be suctioned and cleared. The mouth should be visualized for blood, mucus, or broken teeth (Figure 1-9). The stability of the maxilla and mandible should be confirmed by assessing each bone (Figure 1-10).

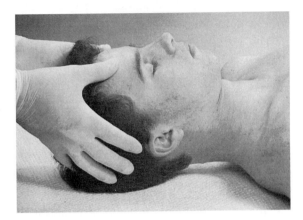

Figure 1-6 Palpate and examine the head for any deformity or bleeding.

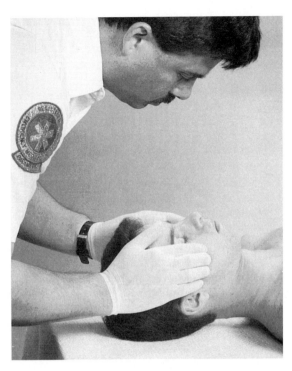

Figure 1-7 All bones of the facial area must be evaluated.

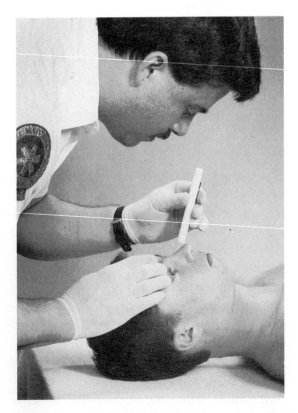

Figure 1-8 Briefly examine the eyes, using a penlight.

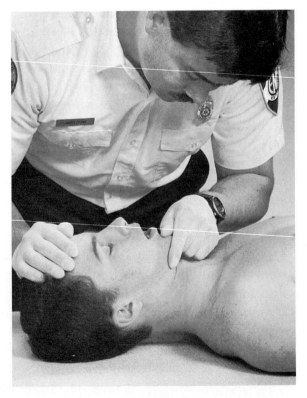

Figure 1-9 The mouth should be examined for blood, mucus, or broken teeth.

</>

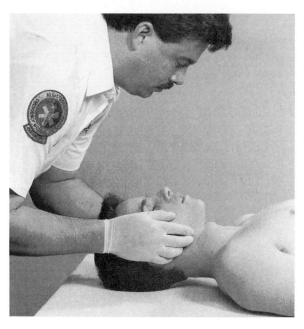

Figure 1-10 Palpate the maxilla and mandible, looking for any abnormalities.

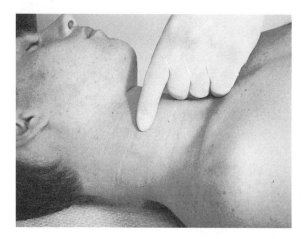

Figure 1-11 Jugular venous distention.

Neck

The neck should be visualized for the presence or absence of jugular venous distention (Figure 1-11). The thyroid cartilage should be midline with the trachea. Tracheal tugging should be absent during respirations. Palpation should note an equal carotid pulse bilaterally, and no tenderness or deformity of the cervical spine should be present (Figure 1-12). If trauma is involved, a cervical collar should be applied at this time.

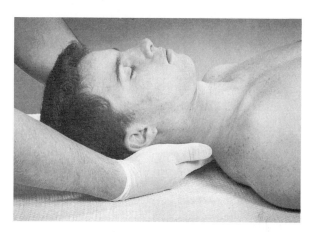

Figure 1-12 Gently palpate the cervical spine.

Upper extremities

A detailed examination of each upper extremity should include palpation for tenderness and deformity, as well as a detailed neurologic and circulatory evaluation. Color, motion, strength, sensitivity, capillary refill, and distal pulses should be evaluated. A bilateral comparison of strength of grip and pushing with the feet provides an excellent method of evaluating each extremity (Figure 1-13). The clavicles are often examined along with the arms, because the humerus articulates at the shoulder.

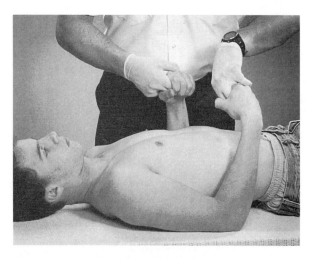

Figure 1-13 Having the patient squeeze your fingers simultaneously will give you a comparison.

Table 1-1 Glasgow Coma Scale	
Response	**Points**
Eye opening	
Spontaneous eye opening	4
Eye opening on command	3
Eye opening to painful stimulus	2
No eye opening	1
Best motor response	
Follows command	6
Localizes painful stimuli*	5
Withdrawal to pain	4
Responds with abnormal flexion to painful stimuli (decorticate)	3
Responds with abnormal extension to pain (decerebrate)	2
Gives no motor response	1
Best verbal response†	
Answers appropriately (oriented)	5
Gives confused answers	4
Inappropriate response	3
Makes unintelligible noises	2
Makes no verbal response	1
TOTAL SCORE:	3-15

The Glasgow Coma Scale, based on eye opening and verbal and motor responses, is a practical means of monitoring changes in level of consciousness. If response on the scale is given a number, the responsiveness of the patient can be expressed by summation of the figures. *Lowest* score is 3, *highest* is 15.
*Apply knuckles to sternum, observe arms.
†Arouse patient with painful stimulus if necessary.

Table 1-2 Trauma Score	
Response	**Points**
Eye opening	
Spontaneous	3
To Voice	2
To Pain	1
None	0
Verbal response	
Oriented	4
Confused	3
Inappropriate words	2
Incomprehensible words	1
None	0
Respiratory effort	
Normal	3
Shallow	1
Retractive	1
None	0
Capillary return	
Normal	2
Delayed	0
Motor responses	
Obeys command	4
Withdraws	3
Flexion	2
Extension	1
None	0
TOTAL SCORE:	

Vital signs

Once the arm is thoroughly evaluated, vital signs should be documented. Blood pressure, pulse, skin condition, capillary refill, and response to pain should be evaluated and documented. Respirations are counted by watching chest movement. Glasgow Coma Scale, Trauma Score, or CRAMS Scale can also be determined at this time (Tables 1-1 to 1-3). Vital signs are reevaluated according to the severity of the patient, which allows the paramedic to note trends or changes in the patient's condition.

Thorax

The anterior and lateral aspects of the thorax are then evaluated. Inspection of the chest should occur first and allows the paramedic to visualize symmetry of the chest wall (Figure 1-14). In addition, signs of developing respiratory distress such as intercostal retractions can be detected. The lungs should be auscultated bilaterally for any remarkable sounds (Figures 1-15 to 1-17; Table 1-4). Breath sounds should be clear and loud bilaterally in the normal patient. Abnormal sounds are summarized in

Text continues on p. 16.

Table 1-3 CRAMS Scale

Response	Points
Circulation	
Normal	2
Abnormal	1
Severely abnormal	0
Respiration	
Normal	2
Abnormal	1
Severely abnormal	0
Abdomen	
Normal	2
Abnormal	1
Severely abnormal	0
Motor	
Normal	2
Abnormal	1
Severely abnormal	0
Speech	
Normal	2
Abnormal	1
Severely abnormal	0
TOTAL SCORE:	

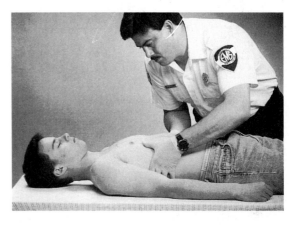

Figure 1-14 Evaluate the chest for symmetry.

Table 1-4 Characteristics of Normal Breath Sounds

Sound	Characteristics	Findings
Vesicular	Heard over most of lung fields; low pitch; soft and short expirations; will be accentuated in a thin person or a child and diminished in the overweight or very muscular	
Bronchovesicular	Heard over main bronchus area and over upper right posterior lung field; medium pitch; expiration equals inspiration	
Bronchial/tracheal	Heard only over trachea; high pitch; loud and long expirations, often somewhat longer than inspiration	

From Seidel HM, Ball JW, Dains JE, et al: Mosby's guide to physical examinations, ed 2, St. Louis, 1991, Mosby; modified from Thompson et al, 1989.

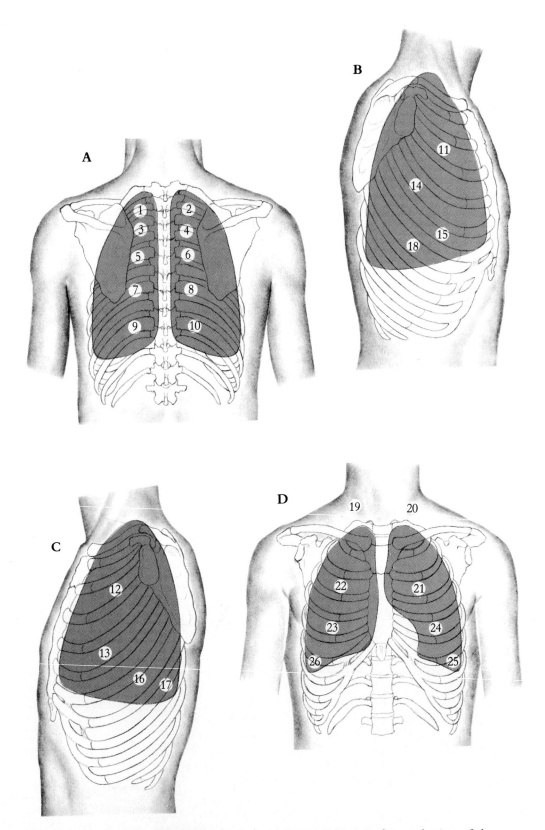

Figure 1-15 Suggested sequence for systematic percussion and auscultation of the thorax. **A,** Posterior thorax. **B,** Right lateral thorax. **C,** Left lateral thorax. **D,** Anterior thorax. (From Seidel HM, Ball JW, Dains JE, et al: *Mosby's guide to physical examination,* ed 2, St. Louis, 1991, Mosby, p 285.)

A

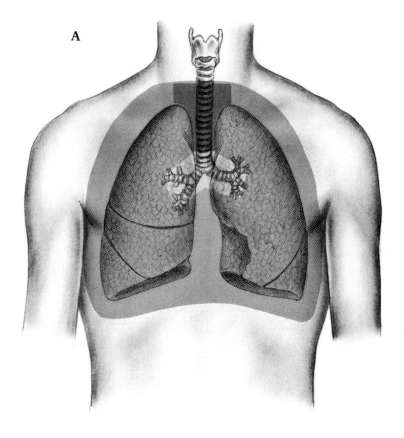

Figure 1-16 Normal auscultatory sounds. **A,** Anterior view. **B,** Posterior view. (From Seidel HM, Ball JW, Dains JE, et al: *Mosby's guide to physical examination,* ed 2, St. Louis, 1991, Mosby, p 288; modified from Thompson JM, et al: *Clinical nursing,* ed 2, St. Louis, 1989, Mosby.)

B

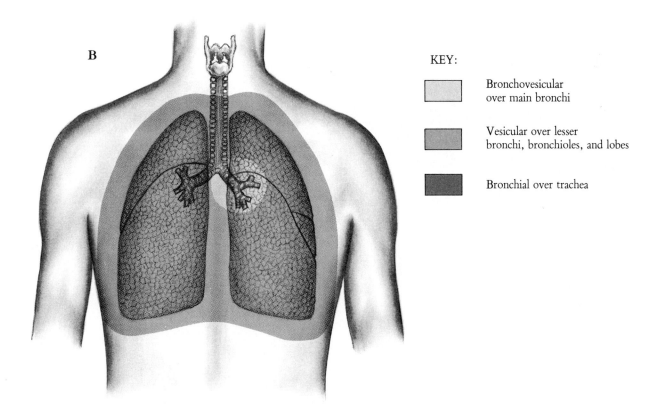

KEY:

Bronchovesicular over main bronchi

Vesicular over lesser bronchi, bronchioles, and lobes

Bronchial over trachea

Figures 1-18 and 1-19. The heart should be auscultated for rate and rhythm; any abnormal sounds such as murmurs or clicks should be noted (Figure 1-20 and Table 1-5). Palpation should include all structures of the thorax: the clavicles, the sternum, and the ribs.

Procedure for auscultating the heart. A routine should be adopted for the various positions the patient is asked to assume, although the paramedic should be prepared to alter the sequence if the patient's condition requires it. The paramedic should instruct the patient when to breathe normally and when to hold the breath in expiration and inspiration. He or she should listen carefully for each heart sound, especially while the respirations are momentarily suspended. The following sequence is suggested:

1. With the patient sitting up and leaning slightly forward, listen in all five areas (see Figure 1-20, *A*). This is the best position to hear the relatively high-pitched murmurs with the stethoscope diaphragm.

2. With the patient supine, listen in all five areas (see Figure 1-20, *B*).

3. With the patient left lateral recumbent, listen in all five areas. This is the best position to hear the low-pitched filling sounds in diastole with the stethoscope bell (see Figure 1-20, *C*).

4. Other positions depend on your findings. If the patient is right lateral recumbent, listen in all five areas. This is the best position for evaluating right rotated heart or dextrocardia.

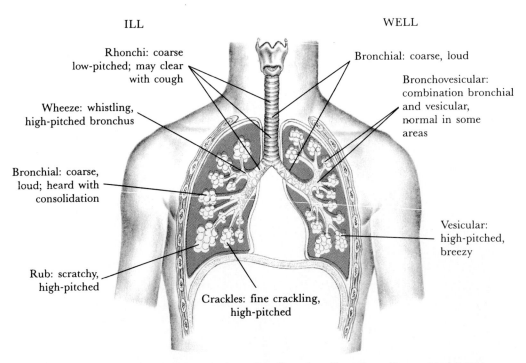

ILL

WELL

Rhonchi: coarse low-pitched; may clear with cough

Wheeze: whistling, high-pitched bronchus

Bronchial: coarse, loud; heard with consolidation

Rub: scratchy, high-pitched

Crackles: fine crackling, high-pitched

Bronchial: coarse, loud

Bronchovesicular: combination bronchial and vesicular, normal in some areas

Vesicular: high-pitched, breezy

Figure 1-17   Schema of breath sounds in the ill and well patient. (From Seidel HM, Ball JW, Dains JE, et al: *Mosby's guide to physical examination,* ed 2, St. Louis, 1991, Mosby, p 289.)

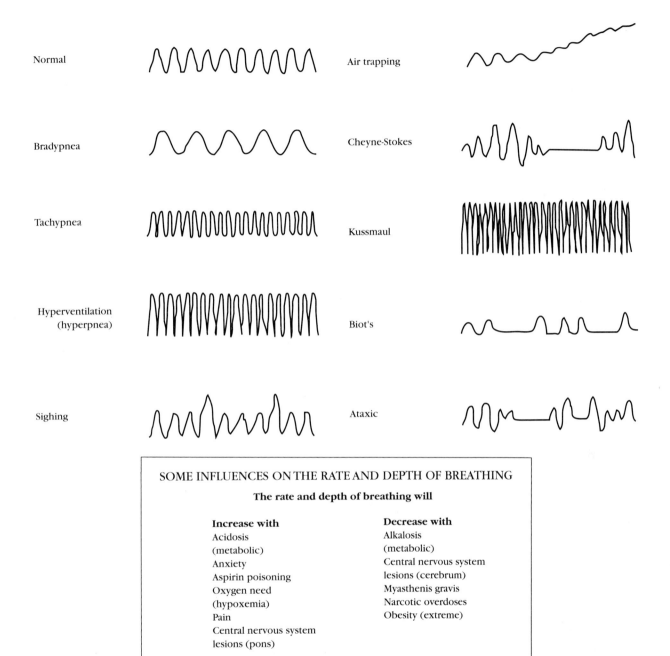

Figure 1-18 Patterns of respiration. The horizontal axis indicates the relative rates of these patterns. The vertical swings of the line drawings indicate the relative depth of respiration. (From Seidel HM, Ball JW, Dains JE, et al: *Mosby's guide to physical examination,* ed 2, St. Louis, 1991, Mosby, p 279.)

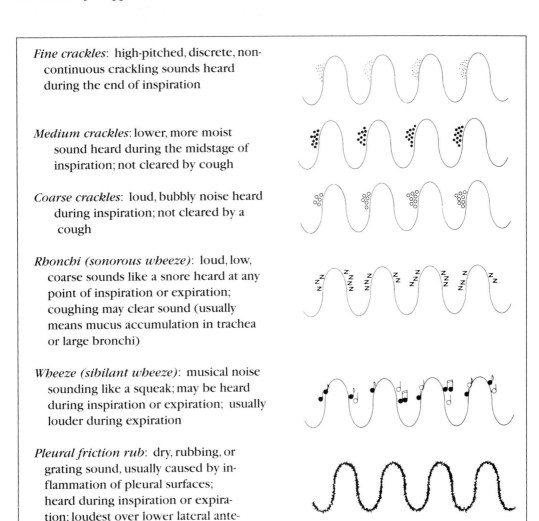

Fine crackles: high-pitched, discrete, non-continuous crackling sounds heard during the end of inspiration

Medium crackles: lower, more moist sound heard during the midstage of inspiration; not cleared by cough

Coarse crackles: loud, bubbly noise heard during inspiration; not cleared by a cough

Rhonchi (sonorous wheeze): loud, low, coarse sounds like a snore heard at any point of inspiration or expiration; coughing may clear sound (usually means mucus accumulation in trachea or large bronchi)

Wheeze (sibilant wheeze): musical noise sounding like a squeak; may be heard during inspiration or expiration; usually louder during expiration

Pleural friction rub: dry, rubbing, or grating sound, usually caused by inflammation of pleural surfaces; heard during inspiration or expiration; loudest over lower lateral anterior surface

Modified from Thompson et al, 1989.

Figure 1-19 Adventitious breath sounds. (From Seidel HM, Ball JW, Dains JE, et al: *Mosby's guide to physical examination,* ed 2, St. Louis, 1991, Mosby, p 291; modified from Thompson JM, et al: *Clinical nursing,* ed 2, St. Louis, 1989, Mosby.)

Abdomen

The abdomen should be visually inspected for any signs of distention or trauma. Contusions are often more serious than they appear and should alert the paramedic to possible underlying injury. Palpation should be performed gently, feeling for abnormal masses or pulsations (Figure 1-21). "Rebound tenderness" should not be elicited in the field, since it gives the paramedic little additional information and may cause the patient unnecessary pain. Similarly, auscultation of the abdomen is rarely considered a field procedure, since it may take up to 10 minutes to perform an examination.

Pelvis and genitalia

The pelvis should be checked for symmetry and stability. Light pressure exerted downward and inward usually suffices in eliciting pain (Figure 1-22). Inspection and palpation may re-

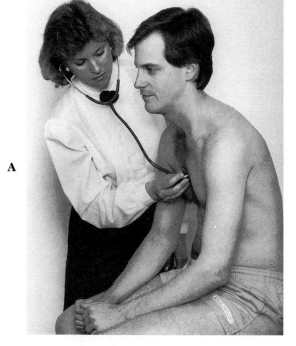

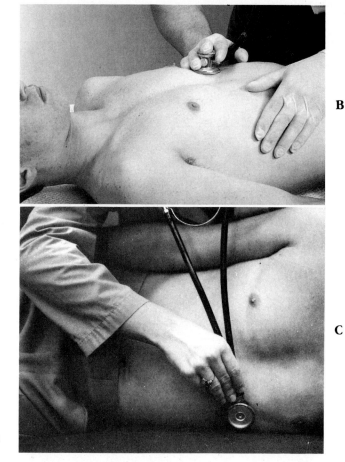

Figure 1-20 Procedure for auscultating the heart: sequence of patient positions for auscultation. **A,** Sitting up, leaning slightly forward. **B,** Supine. **C,** Left lateral recumbent. (**A** and **C** From Malasanos L, Barkauskas V, Stoltenberg-Allen K: *Health Assessment,* ed 4, St. Louis, 1990, Mosby, p 339.)

Table 1-5   Extra Heart Sounds

Sound	Detection	Description
Increased S_3	Bell at apex; patient left lateral recumbent	Early diastole, low pitch
Increased S_4	Bell at apex; patient supine or semilateral	Late diastole or early systole, low pitch
Gallops	Bell at apex; patient supine or left lateral recumbent	Presystole, intense, easily heard
Mitral valve opening snap	Diaphragm medial to apex, may radiate to base; any position, second left intercostal space	Early diastole briefly, before S_3; high pitch, sharp snap or click; not affected by respiration; easily confused with S_2
Systolic clicks	Diaphragm; patient sitting or supine	Late systole, high pitch, intensifies with increased venous return
Aortic valve	Apex, base in second right intercostal space	Early systole, intense, high pitch; radiates; not affected by respirations
Pulmonary valve	Second left intercostal space at sternal border	Early systole, less intense than aortic click; intensifies on expiration, decreases on inspiration
Pericardial friction rub	Widely heard; sound clearest toward apex	May occupy all of systole and diastole; intense, grating, machinelike; may have three components and obliterate heart sounds; if only one or two components, may sound like murmur

veal deformity of the pelvic girdle. Examination of the genitalia should be limited to visualization only. The paramedic should look for any signs of abnormal bleeding or discharge. Priapism may be present in males with spinal cord trauma.

Lower extremities

Examination of the lower extremities should begin with visualization, looking for wounds, edema, or deformities (Figure 1-23). As with the upper extremities, the legs are evaluated for color, motion, strength, sensitivity, capillary refill, and distal pulses (Figure 1-24). An accepted method of assessing the distal neurologic function of the patient is to have the patient push and pull against the palm of your hand. Eliciting a Babinski's reflex by stroking the bottom of the foot is contraindicated if the patient is suspected of having a fracture of the extremity (Figure 1-25).

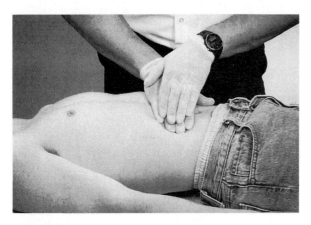

Figure 1-21 Gently palpate the abdomen for tenderness, abnormal masses, or pulsations.

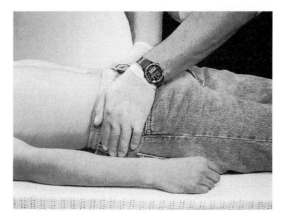

Figure 1-22 Check the pelvis for symmetry and stability by exerting light pressure downward and inward.

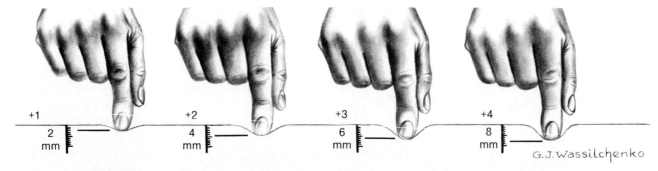

Figure 1-23 Assessing for pitting edema. The severity of edema may be characterized by grading 1+ through 4+. Any concomitant pitting can be mild or severe, as evidenced by the following: 1+, slight pitting, no visible distortion; 2+, a somewhat deeper pit than in 1+, but again no readily detectable distortion; 3+, the pit is noticeably deep, and the dependent extremity looks fuller and swollen; 4+, the pit is very deep, lasts a while, and the dependent extremity is grossly distorted. Note: If edema is unilateral, suspect the occlusion of a major vein. If edema occurs without pitting, suspect arterial disease and occlusion. (From Seidel HM, Ball JW, Dains JE, et al: *Mosby's guide to physical examination,* ed 2, St. Louis, 1991, Mosby, p 355; modified from Canobbia, 1990.)

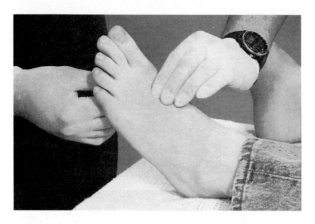

Figure 1-24 The legs are evaluated for color, motion, strength, sensitivity, capillary refill, and distal pulses.

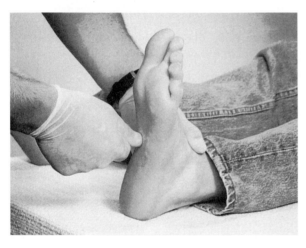

Figure 1-25 Eliciting a Babinski's reflex.

Back

For evaluation of the posterior aspect of the body, the patient must first be correctly positioned. Most medical patients are willing to sit forward to allow the paramedic to examine and listen to their back (Figure 1-26). However, the trauma patient must be logrolled, using spinal precautions (Figure 1-27). Examination of the

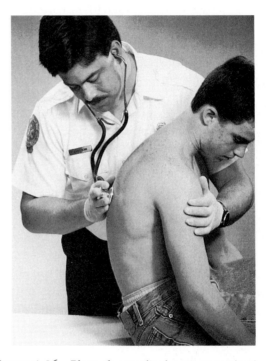

Figure 1-26 Place the medical patient in the forward position to auscultate the posterior chest.

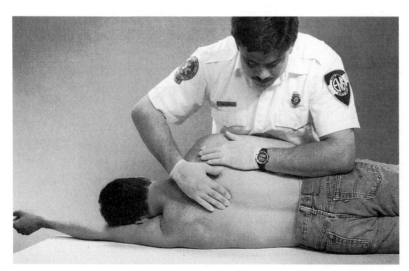

Figure 1-27 Supine patients may be logrolled to examine their back.

A.M.P.L.E.

ALLERGIES: List any allergies that the patient has or anything that may have caused an allergic reaction.

MEDICATIONS: List all medications (prescription and nonprescription) that the patient is currently taking.

PERTINENT PMH: List any pertinent past medical history that is related to the current situation (hospitalizations, injuries, illnesses).

LAST INTAKE: List the last time the patient ate or drank anything. Include a summary of the intake.mh;5q

EVENTS LEADING UP TO AND INCLUDING THE EMERGENCY: Tell what the patient was doing when the current problem developed and how the incident occurred.

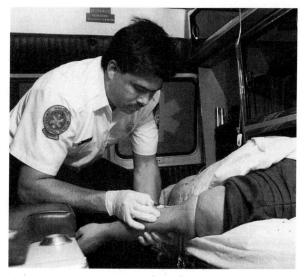

Figure 1-28   Many treatments can be initiated while en route to the hospital.

back and buttocks includes visualization for injuries and ecchymosis; palpation of the spinal column and soft tissue for deformity, muscle guarding, pain, or spasms; and auscultation of the posterior chest.

Past medical history

A patient's *past medical history* is gathered throughout the evaluation. A paramedic should be able to talk with the patient (or family) while performing some of the secondary assessment. During this time, conversation with the patient will elicit important information about the patient's past medical history. The acronym *AMPLE* is used by many to guide them in questioning the patient.

Stage 5: Treatment and Transportation

On completion of the comprehensive assessment, a paramedic should have developed a plan for any additional treatment and stabilization required by the patient. This treatment is known as the *secondary resuscitation*. It is at

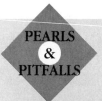

PEARLS
&
PITFALLS

Safety First!

A paramedic is trained to handle most emergency situations. Red lights and sirens (RLSs) are required in only a small percentage of all patients. Transporting patients with minor injuries with RLSs places the patient, the crew, and the public at unnecessary risk for injury, and the crew and EMS organization at increased legal risk. A recent legal settlement of nearly $5 million was reached after a midwestern fire department ambulance broadsided a pickup driven by a 18-year-old female, leaving her partially paralyzed. The patient in the ambulance was being transported to the hospital because of a sprained ankle.

this time that the lesser complaints are addressed, such as minor fractures, lacerations, sprains, or strains. In many EMS systems these types of illnesses or injuries are addressed routinely while en route to the hospital. Treatments such as bandaging, EKG monitoring, and prophylactic IV and drug administration can be easily accomplished in the back of a moving ambulance (Figure 1-28). Decisions regarding transportation to an appropriate facility should be made in accordance with the severity of the patient and local protocols and in consultation with medical control.

Stage 6: Reevaluation

Reevaluation is a continuous process. It must be performed throughout the call, from the first contact and assessment of the patient through the transfer of care for the patient to the next provider (Figure 1-29). A paramedic develops this skill with practice and experience. The reevaluation phase may be the most important factor in caring for the patient, for it is here that decompensation is most often recognized. A paramedic should be aware that anything can happen at anytime with a patient in crisis.

For a reevaluation to provide relevant information, an initial baseline evaluation must have been performed. By comparing the initial findings to those on reevaluation, a more accurate picture can be painted for the paramedic, the medical control physician, and the receiving medical personnel.

◆ Pulling It All Together

Patient evaluation is a process that requires much practice in the classroom and in clinical settings. The learning process allows each paramedic to develop his own style. One way of doing this is to develop a personalized assessment and documentation technique. Many paramedics like to use an assessment method that is similar to their method of documentation. Two of the most common evaluation/documentation techniques are the SOAPIE and CHART methods. These methods allow a paramedic the leeway to evaluate a patient as deemed necessary and still provide for a mechanism of thorough documentation.

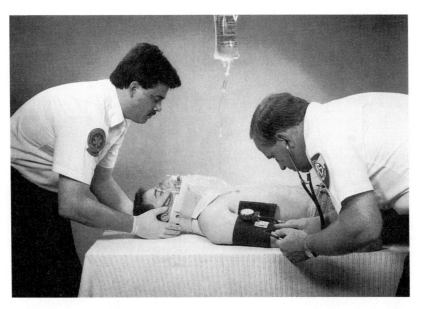

Figure 1-29 Reevaluate the patient often.

S.O.A.P.I.E.

SUBJECTIVE INFORMATION: Information told to you that cannot be obtained by physical examination. The patient's chief complaint, past medical history, medications, symptoms and information from bystanders/family are included in this segment.

OBJECTIVE EXAMINATION: The purpose of the objective examination is to support the information gathered in the subjective segment. Included in this step are the physical examination, vital signs, and all of the data gained by your senses.

ASSESSMENT: The term *assessment* in this context is somewhat misleading. At this point, assessment represents a synthesis of information found in the subjective and objective examination. The paramedic can develop a working field diagnosis or conclusion as to what is possibly wrong with the patient.

PLAN: This phase includes how the paramedic plans to treat the patient. It involves information from medical consultation, as well as actual treatment modalities intended for the patient.

IMPLEMENTATION: This phase is a follow-up of the paramedic's plan for treatment. It includes those treatment modalities that were successful, as well as those that were unsuccessful. It is also important to document the procedures that were not successful for reasons such as proximity to the hospital, battery failure of a defibrillator, or infiltration of an IV site.

EVALUATION: This last step is actually one that occurs throughout your entire contact time with the patient. A continual reevaluation of the patient is most important because it allows the paramedic to redirect treatment modalities according to patient response.

C.H.A.R.T.

CHIEF COMPLAINT: The chief complaint phase includes most of the subjective information that is provided to you by the patient and family. Direct quotations made by the patient such as, "This is the worst pain I've ever had," and why the ambulance was called are extremely valuable in this segment.

HISTORY (HX): The remainder of the subjective information is included in this section of the patient evaluation. It should include the patient's age, weight, general appearance, and a summary of the current problem. Pertinent past medical history that is related to the chief complaint should also be included here.

ASSESSMENT: Information gathered from your objective evaluation is noted here. The specifics of your primary and secondary evaluations are detailed, as well as Glasgow Coma and Trauma scores.

RX (TREATMENT): An overview of the care given to the patient should be noted, including a response to that treatment. Remember to document even those procedures that were attempted but not completed, as well as any complications incurred.

TRANSPORTATION: All information concerning the patient's transport to the hospital is documented at this time. This is an opportunity to summarize the mode of transport to the hospital, any changes noted in reevaluation of the patient, and any additional treatment modalities rendered.

Testing Your Knowledge

1. List the six stages of patient evaluation.

2. The first step in performing a primary survey is to evaluate the patient's:

    a. Responsiveness.
    b. Airway status.
    c. Circulatory status.
    d. Vital signs.

3. The paramedic may obtain patient information from which of the following sources?

    a. The patient
    b. First responders
    c. Family members
    d. All of the above

4. The primary survey is conducted to elicit which of the following?

    a. Cervical spine injuries
    b. Signs of trauma
    c. Life-threatening emergencies
    d. Nonlife-threatening emergencies

5. Explain the A,B,C,D,E plan for performing a primary survey.

6. Define airway patency.

7. On removal of a victim from a burning building, which of the following is *NOT* an appropriate question to ask regarding the history of the fire?

    a. What was the nature of the combusted material?
    b. Was the fire arson or accidentally set?
    c. Did the patient lose consciousness?
    d. How long was the patient exposed?

8. From the following list, select the one that *BEST* exemplifies a chief complaint.

    a. "The pain started yesterday."
    b. BP = 200/110
    c. "I've been on heart pills for 2 years."
    d. "I feel like I'm going to throw up."

9. The paramedic is responsible for:

    a. Carefully evaluating the patient's vital signs and symptoms.
    b. Providing prompt and appropriate emergency medical care.
    c. Providing safe transportation to a medical facility.
    d. All of the above.

10. From the following list, select the one which **BEST** exemplifies objective information.

    a. Nausea
    b. Diaphoresis
    c. Headache
    d. Thirst

11. In performing a primary survey, the paramedic must inspect both the anterior and posterior aspect of the body.

    a. True
    b. False

12. Generally speaking, in the case of a critical patient, the paramedic might not exit the primary resuscitation phase of treatment.

    a. True
    b. False

13. What do the letters A-V-P-U represent?

14. What does the acronym AMPLE represent?

15. On the basis of the case scenario at the beginning of this chapter, write patient reports based on the SOAPIE and CHART methods of documentation.

Answers are in Appendix A.

Patient Evaluation

The patient evaluation should take no longer than 10 minutes to complete. The paramedic should communicate with the patient at all times and should render treatment when appropriate. Failure to render care will result in not being awarded points.

Primary and secondary surveys and resuscitation	Possible points	Points awarded
Primary survey		
Evaluate scene, safety, and mechanism of injury for possible cervical spine involvement.	1	
Open airway while protecting cervical spine and continue to monitor patency at all times.	1	
Check for breathing and quick chest examination (anterior and posterior) for chest trauma. Breathes for patient if not adequate and corrects any life-threatening chest injury. Oxygen is applied appropriate to injury.	2	
Check circulation and major bleeding. (Evaluate strength and approximate rate of pulse, perform quick body scan to identify gross bleeding). Correct any life-threatening problems found.	3	
Evaluate skin condition for color, moisture, and turgor.	1	
Perform mini-neurologic evaluation (AVPU).	1	
Expose and examine any area of body for life-threatening illness/injury not yet performed.	1	
Secondary survey		
Inspect and palpate head and face for deformity and bleeding, without moving cervical spine.	1	
Examine eyes, ears and mouth. Note presence/absence of Battle's sign.	4	
Examine neck for midline trachea and jugular vein distention. Gently palpate cervical spine for deformity and tenderness. Apply cervical collar (if suggested).	3	
Examine upper extremities for injury. Evaluate strength, color, motion, sensitivity, capillary refill, and pulses. Clavicle may be included.	4	
Evaluate vital signs (BP, HR, RR minimum).	3	
Inspect and auscultate chest. Identify equal, bilateral chest expansion.	2	
Inspect and palpate the abdomen (four quadrants).	2	
Palpate pelvic arches, check for priapism in males with suspected spinal trauma.	1	
Examine lower extremities for injury. Evaluate strength, color, motion, sensitivity, capillary refill, and pulses.	4	
Logroll and examine back for deformity, bleeding, and signs of ecchymosis.	1	
Re-evaluate vital signs (BP, HR, RR).	3	
SUBTOTAL FROM PRIMARY	10	
SUBTOTAL FROM SECONDARY	28	
TOTAL SCORE	38	

BIBLIOGRAPHY

Ball RA: Documentation—the overlooked aspect of emergency care, *J Emerg Med Serv* 15(5):31-32, 1990.

Bledsoe BE, Porter RS, Shade BR, et al: *Paramedic emergency care*, Englewood Cliffs, NJ, 1991, Brady Publishing (Prentice-Hall).

Canan S, Seaver J: Little habits that could save you, *J Emerg Med Serv* 16(4):37, 1991.

Caroline NL: *Emergency care in the streets*, ed 3, Boston, 1987, Little, Brown.

Clawson J: Running hot and the case of Sharron Rose, *J Emerg Med Serv* 16(7):11-13, 1991.

Dick T: Putting it into words, *J Emerg Med Serv* 12(12):26-28, 1987.

Krebs DR, Henry KC, Gabriele MB: *When violence erupts—a survival guide for emergency responders*, St. Louis, 1990, Mosby.

Seidel HM, Ball JW, Bains JE et al: *Mosby's guide to physical assessment*, St. Louis, 1991, Mosby.

Shade BR: Documentation of information-protection for the EMT, *Emer Magazine* 17(4):32-35, 1985.

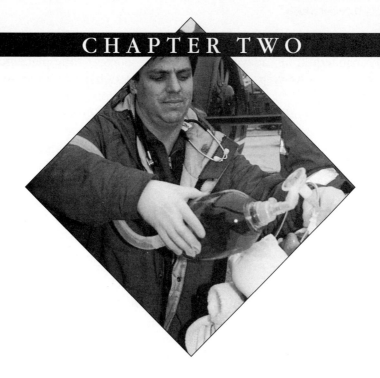

CHAPTER TWO

Advanced Airway Management

Objectives

A paramedic should be able to—

1. Given an unlabeled diagram of the airway, identify the key anatomic structures.

2. Given four types of esophageal airways, identify the key features and two advantages of each device (EOA, EGTA, PTL, and ETC).

3. List three indications and contra-indications for each of the airways listed in Objective 2.

4. List three indications for endotracheal intubation.

5. Discuss two situations when nasotracheal intubation may be more advantageous than orotracheal intubation.

6. Define and differentiate between the two major types of laryngoscope blades.

7. Given various scenarios, explain how the prehospital provider determines which laryngoscope blade to use for each situation.

8. Discuss two situations in which digital intubation may be indicated.

9. Define and list three indications for performing a cricothyrotomy.

10. List five complications of a cricothyrotomy.

11. Define and list five complications of percutaneous transtracheal ventilation.

12. List three potential side effects or hazards of suctioning.

13. Using an airway mannequin or cadaver model, demonstrate the following procedures:
   a. Proper insertion and ventilation using the various types of endotracheal airways
   b. Proper endotracheal intubation and ventilation technique
   c. Proper nasotracheal intubation and ventilation technique
   d. Proper technique for determining correct tube placement for both the esophageal airway devices and the endotracheal tube
   e. Proper technique for performing a needle and a surgical cricothyrotomy
   f. Proper technique for suctioning of the nonintubated and the tracheally intubated patient
   g. Proper technique for retrieval of a foreign body from the airway using direct laryngoscopy

Photo courtesy Michael Kowal/Journal of Emergency Medical Services.

Case Scenario

3:07 AM   You are dispatched as a paramedic assist with the local fire department to a residential fire in a geriatric retirement community just west of town. A townhome is found engulfed in flames, with smoke billowing from the eaves. The fire fighters have just carried out an elderly female from the building, and they place her directly into your unit. In performing your primary assessment, you determine that the patient is not breathing and begin to hyperventilate her with a bag-valve-mask (BVM) device and high-concentration oxygen. She has a rapid pulse in both the carotid and radial arteries. Body survey notes no obvious injuries or burns.

After approximately 2 minutes, the patient still is not breathing, and her EKG now shows some ventricular ectopy. Pulse oximetry shows an SaO$_2$ of 91%. The decision is made to endotracheally intubate the patient. A 7.5-mm endotracheal tube is selected and lubricated with water-soluble jelly. Following continued hyperventilation, direct laryngoscopy is performed. A small amount of secretion is seen in front of the vocal cords, making visualization difficult. The patient is suctioned, using a tonsil-tip suction catheter. Following reventilation, direct laryngoscopy is performed, and the endotracheal tube (ETT) is passed without difficulty; the bulb is inflated with 5 cc of air. Breath sounds are confirmed bilaterally; however, wheezes are noted in all fields. Ventilations are continued at a rate of 20 breaths/minute.

While en route to the hospital, the patient begins to breathe on her own, and much of the wheezing is diminished. Upon presentation to the emergency department staff, approximately 10 minutes following your initial intervention, the patient is now awake, responds to your voice, shows an EKG of sinus rhythm with a rate of 90 beats per minute, and pulse oximetry of 96%. You explain to her what has happened, where she is, and why she is unable to speak.

Following a brief hospital stay for additional evaluation and monitoring, the patient is discharged.

Death caused by airway compromise is an ancient phenomenon. Even prehistoric man must have stood helpless watching his friends die from choking; later he probably felt the frustration of failure as he attempted to devise ways of saving them.

The Bible tells of the Prophet Elisha resuscitating a young lad with mouth-to-mouth respiration. The young boy, it seems, collapsed after complaining of a headache. Ancient Egyptians discovered that occasionally life could be restored by breathing into a person's body. In the year 100 BC, Asclepiades, a Greek surgeon, apparently performed the first tracheostomy. The first definite account of tracheostomy was recorded by Musa Brassarolo of Ferrara in 1546. The search for an ideal airway has continued since then. It wasn't until 1880, when McEwen described inserting vulcanite tubes into the trachea, that research toward finding better means of airway control took a different direction.

The advent of Emergency Medical Services (EMSs) in the last two decades has caused a rapid surge in the quest for a better and simpler airway. Numerous options are available to gain airway control. These depend on the rescuer's level of training and local protocols. This section describes the various choices that are available to the EMS provider. Not all of these skills may be allowed in an EMS system. Variations in local protocols may occur.

Before attempting to gain airway control by advanced skills, it is important to oxygenate the patient using basic techniques. Apneic patients may need mouth-to-mask or BVM ventilation while preparation is being made for advanced airway management. Quite often, proper oxygenation, along with oral or nasopharyngeal airway insertion, may be all that is necessary to manage the airway. Should these measures prove inadequate, endotracheal intubation should be the next step. When endotracheal intubation is not feasible, emergency medical technicians (EMTs)/paramedics in some parts of the nation are trained to use either percutaneous transtracheal ventilation (needle cricothyrotomy) or cricothyrotomy (surgical cricothyrotomy).

Aggressive airway management is one of the primary responsibilities of an advanced life support provider. Management begins by recognizing when an advanced procedure is needed.

The paramedic has many options in determining which procedure or device is best for the patient in a particular situation. In this chapter on advanced airway management, the following procedures are discussed:

- Airways using the esophageal principle
  - Esophageal obturator airway
  - Esophageal gastric tube airway
  - Pharyngeal tracheal lumen airway
  - Esophageal tracheal combitube
- Endotracheal intubation
- Nasotracheal intubation

> ### Indications for Advanced Airway Management
>
> - Cardiorespiratory arrest
> - Coma
> - Impending respiratory failure
> - Partial or complete airway obstruction
> - Trauma (direct or indirect)
> - Altered level of consciousness
> - Systemic infections (sepsis)
> - Allergic reaction or anaphylaxis
> - Respiratory paralysis

- Insertion of a large-bore needle through the cricothyroid membrane
- Surgical airway such as the cricothyrotomy or tracheostomy
- Advanced suctioning

◆ Airways Using Esophageal Obturator Principle

Esophageal Obturator Airway
Background

The esophageal obturator airway (EOA) was first described by Don Michael in 1968. The principle is simple: the esophagus is occluded by passing a cuffed, blind-ended tube into it. This prevents the air delivered in the hypopharynx from entering the stomach. A tight-fitting mask is needed to ensure adequate air delivery into the pharynx, larynx, trachea, and lungs and to prevent air from escaping through the mouth and the nose. This technique is extremely simple and has been used extensively in various EMS systems.

The EOA is a large-bore tube with a blind distal end. The tube is 37 cm (16 inches) long and is fitted with a large-volume (35 cc) cuff distally. The tube is fitted through a cuffed, clear facemask. It has 16 openings at the level of the pharynx. The cuff around the mask ensures proper face seal in the hands of a trained ventilator.

Indications

- Deep coma, cardiac and/or respiratory arrest
- When endotracheal intubation is not possible or available
- When BVM ventilation is not adequate or is causing excessive gastric distention

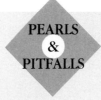

PEARLS & PITFALLS

Advantages and Disadvantages of the EOA

Advantages

- It is easy to insert the airway. The tube is blindly inserted into the esophagus. No direct lower airway visualization is required.
- It prevents aspiration of stomach contents.
- Less training time is required, coupled with greater success rate of insertion by the EMS providers than endotracheal intubation.
- Insertion is possible without extending the neck.

Disadvantages

- An absolutely tight facemask seal is essential. This is difficult to accomplish during patient transport.
- The tube may be introduced inadvertently into the trachea, thereby causing total airway obstruction or damage from the inflated 35-cc cuff.
- Because the esophagus is occluded, pressure may build up in the stomach and the esophagus during retching, resulting in esophageal rupture.
- Upper airway secretions may enter the trachea, since the esophagus is occluded, causing aspiration.
- Excessive cuff inflation may cause pressure necrosis and damage to the esophagus.
- The tube is not anchored to the patient; accidental dislodgement during transport may cause injury to the esophagus.

Contraindications

- Patients with an intact gag reflex
- Facial trauma, especially with facial fractures and/or significant bleeding into the airway
- Esophageal trauma
- Suspected foreign body airway obstruction
- Children under 16 years of age
- Anyone less than 5 feet in height
- Patients taller than 6 feet, 7 inches
- Ingestion of caustic substance
- Esophageal varices
- Cirrhosis of the liver
- Suspected chronic alcohol abuse

Procedure

See p. 33.

Esophageal Gastric Tube Airway
Background

The esophageal gastric tube airway (EGTA) is a modified EOA. Instead of a blind or closed end, the tube has a lumen throughout its length, permitting the passage of a gastric tube to empty the stomach contents. There are no air holes in the tube itself. Ventilation is carried out through a separate opening in the mask (Figure 2-1).

Indications

- Deep coma, cardiac and/or respiratory arrest
- When endotracheal intubation is not possible or available
- When BVM ventilation is not adequate or is causing excessive gastric distention

Contraindications

- Patients with an intact gag reflex
- Facial trauma, especially with facial fractures and/or significant bleeding into the airway
- Esophageal trauma
- Suspected foreign body airway obstruction
- Children under 16 years of age
- Anyone less than 5 feet in height

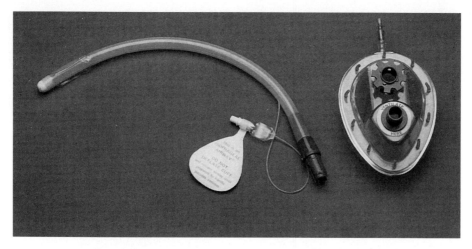

Figure 2-1 Esophageal gastric tube airway (EGTA).

- Patients taller than 6 feet, 7 inches
- Ingestion of caustic substance
- Esophageal varices
- Cirrhosis of the liver
- Suspected chronic alcohol abuse

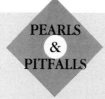

PEARLS & PITFALLS

Advantages and Disadvantages of the EGTA

Advantages
- This modification of the EOA achieves effective stomach decompression and helps to prevent the potential danger of pressure buildup and esophageal rupture.

Disadvantages
- The problem of upper airway secretions, possibly causing aspiration, is not addressed.
- There is the potential danger of total airway obstruction from inadvertent unrecognized tracheal intubation.

Equipment
- EOA or EGTA with appropriate facemask
- Water-soluble lubricant
- BVM
- Oxygen
- 35-cc syringe
- Stethoscope
- Gloves
- Goggles

Procedure (EOA and EGTA)

The technique of insertion is similar for both the tubes. Since there are no air vents in EGTA, ventilation is carried out using a separate port in the mask. Thus the airway essentially is a facemask with the added advantage of esophageal occlusion. In the following section, insertion of EGTA will be described in detail. Differences between EOA and EGTA will be noted.

1. Observe universal precautions. Make sure that the patient is hyperoxygenated by BVM while preparing to insert the EGTA/EOA (Figure 2-2).

2. Attach the tube to the mask and test the cuffs for air leaks (Figures 2-3 and 2-4). The figures show EGTA. The procedure is the same for EOA.

3. Deflate the cuff and lubricate the tube, using a water-soluble lubricant.

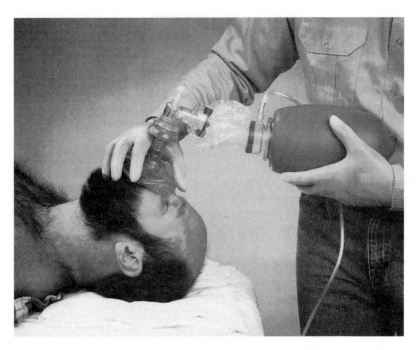

Figure 2-2   Ventilate the patient with a BVM.

4. Hold the head of the patient in the neutral position. Grasp the tongue and jaw with a gloved hand and pull forward. With the other hand, insert the tube through the mouth and into the esophagus. **DO NOT EXTEND THE NECK** (Figure 2-5).

5. Advance the tube gently until the mask rests on the face. The tube is more likely to enter the esophagus than the trachea. When inserted properly, the cuff in the esophagus will be below the level of the carina (Figure 2-6).

6. Fit a ventilating bag onto the mask and deliver two or three positive pressure ventilations. The EOA has only one port on the mask. The EGTA has two ports. The ventilating port is well marked on the mask. A standard 15-mm ventilating bag adapter will not fit over the proximal opening of the tube and its corresponding port.

If the tube has correctly entered the esophagus, the chest will rise. If the tube has been inserted into the trachea, the chest will not rise. Make sure that you auscultate over both lung fields, as well as over the stomach (Figure 2-7). In noisy surroundings such as those usu-

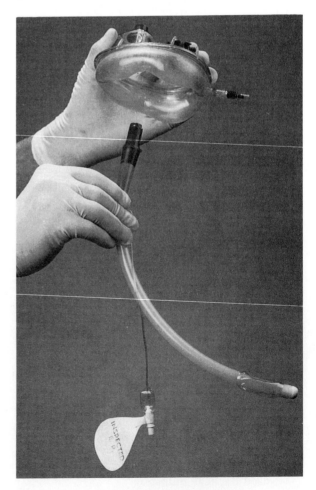

Figure 2-3   Attach the tube to the mask.

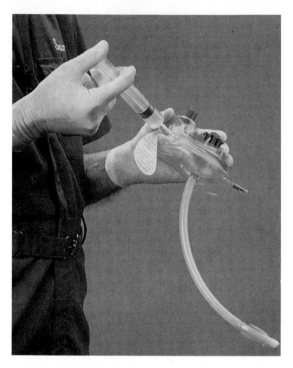

Figure 2-4 Test the cuff.

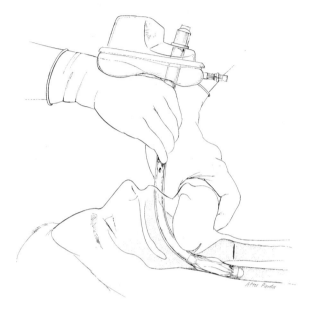

Figure 2-5 Grasp the tongue and jaw and pull forward, inserting the EGTA into the esophagus.

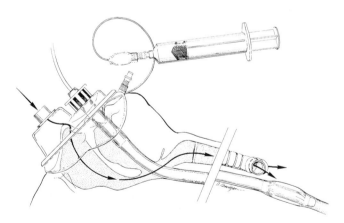

Figure 2-6 Note that the cuff of the EGTA in the esophagus rests below the carina. The posterior wall of the trachea is soft and pliable. If the cuff exerts pressure on the trachea, there is danger of airway occlusion.

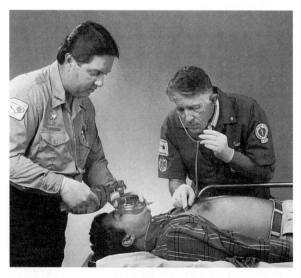

Figure 2-7 Auscultate for breath and epigastric sounds.

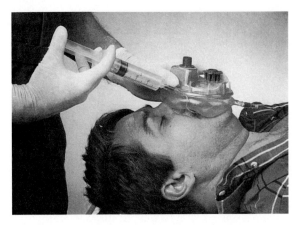

Figure 2-8 Inflate the cuff with 30 to 35 cc of air.

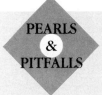

Procedural Problems

- If difficulty is encountered while advancing the tube, pull back slightly. Pull the jaw and tongue forward and slightly toward the feet, and try advancing again. If there is still difficulty, abandon the procedure.
- The EOA/EGTA is a temporary device. As soon as possible, an ETT should be inserted. It is not necessary to remove the EOA/EGTA once intubation has occurred in the field. However, it is recommended that the EOA/EGTA should not be left in place for more than 2 hours.
- Do not remove the EOA/EGTA until the trachea is intubated and the ETT cuff is inflated. Removal of the tube may precipitate regurgitation of stomach contents into the oropharynx, posing threat of aspiration. In the event the tube must be removed before endotracheal intubation (e.g., when the patient starts to regain consciousness and gags on the tube), make sure you have suction equipment handy. Be prepared to turn the patient on his or her side (logroll if necessary).

ally encountered in the field or in the ambulance, it is easy to mistake transmitted sounds from the stomach as "breath sounds."

7. After making sure of proper tube position, inflate the cuff with 30 to 35 of air (Figure 2-8).

8. Reconfirm the placement of the device by listening to the breath sounds bilaterally, making sure that no gurgling sounds are heard over the epigastrium.

9. Ventilate the patient and monitor adequacy of ventilation closely.

10. Make sure suction is available during and after the procedure.

11. Limit movement of the mask and the tube to minimize the risk of esophageal damage.

Pharyngeal Tracheal Lumen Airway
Background

In the search for simple but safer airways for prehospital use, the pharyngeal tracheal lumen (PTL) airway has drawn considerable attention. Endotracheal intubation continues to be the procedure of choice for airway control, but the PTL attempts to address some of the disadvantages of the EOA and EGTA.

The PTL has two parallel tubes of unequal length. The longer tube is 31 cm in overall length; the shorter tube measures 21 cm. The longer tube has a distal cuff (for esophageal or tracheal occlusion). The short tube has a large cuff just proximal to its end (for upper airway occlusion). The long tube measures approximately 22 cm from the teeth strap (Figure 2-9).

The airway is inserted until the teeth strap fits against the incisors. The cuffs are then inflated simultaneously by blowing into the port containing a one-way valve. The rescuer attempts ventilation through the short tube (pharyngeal lumen). The chest will rise if the long tube is in the esophagus. Ventilation is then carried out through the short tube. In this mode, it essentially acts as an EGTA. However,

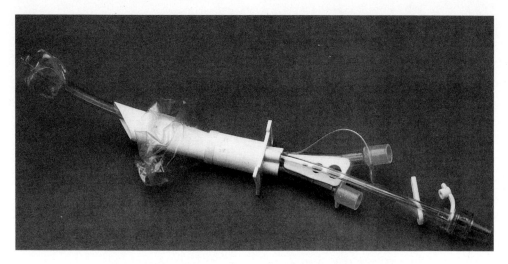

Figure 2-9 Pharyngeal tracheal lumen (PTL) airway.

no facemask is necessary because the large cuff occludes the pharynx proximally.

If the long tube has entered the trachea, blowing air into the short tube will **NOT** cause the chest to rise. Ventilation is then attempted through the long tube, and tracheal placement is confirmed. The large proximal cuff is then deflated. In this mode the tube acts as an ETT.

Indications

◆ Deep coma, cardiac and/or respiratory arrest
◆ When endotracheal intubation is not possible or available
◆ When BVM ventilation is not adequate or is causing excessive gastric distention

Contraindications

◆ Patients with an intact gag reflex
◆ Facial and/or esophageal trauma
◆ Suspected foreign body airway obstruction
◆ Children under 16 years of age
◆ Anyone less than 5 feet in height

Equipment

◆ PTL airway
◆ Water-soluble lubricant
◆ BVM
◆ Oxygen
◆ Stethoscope
◆ Gloves
◆ Goggles

Procedure

1. Observe universal precautions.

2. Ensure adequate oxygenation while preparing to insert the PTL.

3. Test the cuffs on the PTL. Familiarize yourself with the various tubings in the airway. Identify the long and the short tube before insertion.

4. Lubricate the tube with water-soluble jelly.

5. Grasp the patient's tongue and jaw with your gloved left hand and pull forward (Figure 2-10).

6. Gently insert the airway, advancing it until the teeth strap fits against the incisors.

7. Inflate both balloons simultaneously by blowing into the valve (Figure 2-11).

8. Ventilate the patient through the short tube (Figure 2-12). Look for the chest to rise and listen to the breath sounds.

9. *IF THE CHEST RISES,* continue ventilation through the short tube. A gastric tube may be inserted through the long tube, the tip of which is in the esophagus (Figure 2-13). Secure the teeth strap firmly with adhesive tape.

10. *IF THE CHEST DOES NOT RISE,* attempt ventilation through the long tube to check to

PEARLS & PITFALLS

Advantages and Disadvantages of the PTL

The technique of insertion is very similar to that of EOA. However, the training time for PTL insertion is less than that required for endotracheal intubation.

Advantages

* Ventilation is possible, irrespective of tracheal or esophageal placement.
* The proximal cuff prevents blood, secretions, and tissue from being aspirated into the trachea.
* In the "esophageal obturator mode," gastric contents can be suctioned out by inserting a gastric tube through the long tube of the PTL (EGTA offers this advantage also).
* There is no need for a facemask.

Disadvantages

* The PTL is a complicated and cumbersome-looking device. The EMS provider must become thoroughly familiar with the tube, since it can be intimidating.
* In the esophageal mode, the distal cuff will be at a level proximal to the carina (most adults measure 25 to 28 cm from the incisors to the carina). There is a danger of pressure against the posterior trachea with occlusion of the tracheal lumen.
* The procedure is blind. It should not be used in suspected foreign body airway obstruction.
* Even though it is not necessary to extend the neck for insertion of the tube, in actual practice some manipulation of the neck may be necessary to guide the tube into the pharynx.

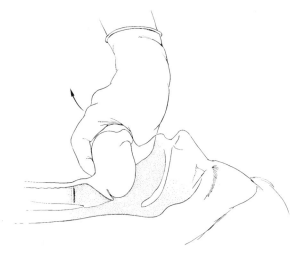

Figure 2-10 Grasp the patient's tongue and jaw and pull forward.

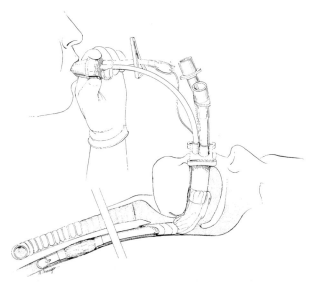

Figure 2-11 Inflate both balloons simultaneously by blowing into the valve.

see if it has entered the trachea. The chest should rise. Continue ventilation through the long tube (Figure 2-14). The proximal cuff may now be deflated. You have **ENDOTRACHE-ALLY** intubated the patient successfully.

Esophageal Tracheal Combitube
Background

Like the PTL, the esophageal tracheal combitube (ETC) has drawn considerable attention

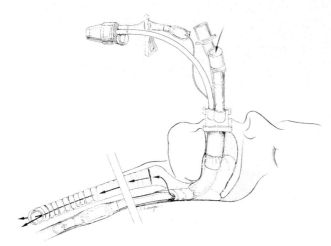

Figure 2-12 Ventilate the patient through the short tube.

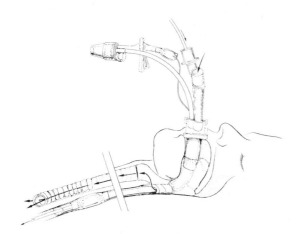

Figure 2-13 *IF THE CHEST RISES,* a gastric tube may be inserted through the long tube into the esophagus and stomach.

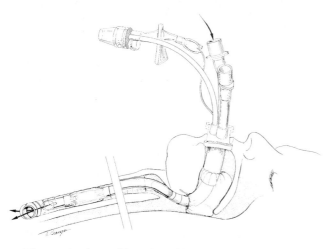

Figure 2-14 *IF THE CHEST DOES NOT RISE,* attempt ventilation through the long tube.

in the search for simple but safer airways for prehospital use. It, too, attempts to address some of the disadvantages of the EOA and the EGTA. The ETC is a twin-lumen plastic tube. One lumen resembles an EOA with a blind distal end. The other looks like an ETT.

The ETC has two balloons: a large proximal balloon and a smaller distal balloon. The tube is inserted blindly. Ventilation can be carried out irrespective of whether the tube enters the esophagus or the trachea.

Indications

◆ Deep coma, cardiac and/or respiratory arrest
◆ When endotracheal intubation is not possible or available
◆ When BVM ventilation is not adequate or is causing excessive gastric distention

Contraindications

◆ Patients with an intact gag reflex
◆ Facial and/or esophageal trauma
◆ Suspected foreign body airway obstruction
◆ Children under 16 years of age
◆ Anyone less than 5 feet in height

Equipment

◆ ETC airway
◆ Water-soluble lubricant
◆ BVM
◆ Stethoscope
◆ Gloves
◆ Goggles

Procedure

1. Observe universal precautions.
2. Ensure adequate oxygenation while preparing to insert the ETC.
3. Test the cuffs on the ETC. Familiarize yourself with the various tubings in the airway. Identify the long and the short tube before insertion.
4. Lubricate the tube with water-soluble jelly.

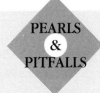

Advantages and Disadvantages of the ETC

Advantages

* In the esophageal mode, stomach contents can be aspirated through the open-ended tube, preventing gastric distention and rupture.
* There is no need for a facemask. The large proximal balloon provides a tight seal in the pharynx. It is claimed that the seal provided by the ETC is better than that of the PTL.
* The danger of unrecognized tracheal intubation is said to be minimal, since ventilation is possible with either esophageal or tracheal placement.
* The design is somewhat simpler than that of the PTL.
* The proximal large cuff is located slightly posteriorly compared to PTL. This may cause better obstruction of the pharynx by pressing the uvula against the nasopharynx.

Disadvantages

* The disadvantages and the technique of insertion of the ETC are the same as those of the PTL.

5. Grasp the patient's tongue and jaw with your gloved left hand and pull forward.

6. Gently insert the airway, advancing it until the printed ring is aligned with the teeth.

7. Inflate line 1 (blue pilot balloon) leading to the pharyngeal cuff with 100 cc of air. (The ETC is packaged with a 140-cc syringe for this purpose.)

8. Inflate line 2 (white pilot balloon) leading to the distal cuff with approximately 15 cc of air. (The ETC is packaged with a 20-cc syringe for this purpose.)

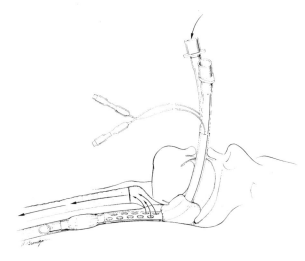

Figure 2-15 When properly placed, the ETC is in the esophagus. Ventilate the patient through the long tube.

9. Ventilate the patient through the longer blue tube (Figure 2-15). Look for the chest to rise and listen to the breath and epigastric sounds.

10. *IF THE CHEST RISES AND EPIGASTRIC SOUNDS ARE NEGATIVE,* continue ventilation through the blue tube. A gastric tube may be inserted through the short tube, the tip of which is in the esophagus. The device is secured by the 100-cc pharyngeal cuff.

11. *IF THE CHEST DOES NOT RISE AND EPIGASTRIC SOUNDS ARE POSITIVE,* attempt ventilation through the shorter, clear tube, to check to see if it has entered the trachea (Figure 2-16). The chest should rise. Continue ventilation through the shorter tube. You have **ENDOTRACHEALLY** intubated the patient successfully.

♦ Endotracheal Intubation

Orotracheal Intubation

Background

Despite recent advances in the search for superior, acceptable, and safer airway control, for over a century endotracheal intubation has remained the "gold standard" for securing and maintaining a compromised airway.

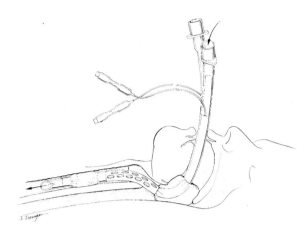

Figure 2-16 If the ETC is placed into the trachea, ventilate the patient through the short tube.

Endotracheal intubation is a skill that is mastered only after many hours of competent training and practice. If not used frequently, the skill can rapidly deteriorate. The EMS provider should be aware of this and take proper measures to maintain a high level of competence. The skill can be taught using mannequins, cadavers, or anesthetized patients in the operating room.

Indications

◆ Coma, respiratory and/or cardiac arrest
◆ Impending airway obstruction/respiratory failure (e.g., burns to the airway, severe asthma, chronic obstructive pulmonary disease [COPD]) exacerbation, severe pulmonary edema when the patient develops fatigue and may go into respiratory arrest)
◆ Patients without a gag reflex who need gastric lavage should be intubated first to prevent aspiration (e.g., drug overdose, bleeding in the gastrointestinal tract)
◆ When prolonged artificial ventilation is required

Contraindication

◆ When attempts at intubation could precipitate laryngospasm

Advantages and Disadvantages of Endotracheal Intubation

Advantages

◆ Endotracheal intubation provides definitive airway control, unlike the esophageal airways, which must be replaced by an ETT as soon as possible.
◆ It involves direct visualization. There is no danger of blindly pushing an obstructing foreign body farther down into the airway.
◆ It provides a tight seal to the trachea so that there is no danger of aspiration of stomach contents.
◆ Unlike cricothyrotomy or tracheostomy, advanced surgical skills are not needed.
◆ ETT placement provides an alternate route for medication administration. The acronym NAVEL is used to indicate medications that can be given via ETT: Narcan (naloxone), atropine, Valium (diazepam), epinephrine, and lidocaine.

Disadvantages

◆ Skill deterioration may occur without frequent field intubations or practice with mannequins.
◆ Despite direct visualization of the trachea, esophageal intubation may occur. Sometimes this is hard to detect, especially in noisy surroundings.
◆ In victims of multiple trauma, it may be difficult to maintain cervical spine immobilization and insert the ETT at the same time.
◆ The procedure may produce retching, vomiting, increase in intracranial pressure, or cardiac dysrhythmias.

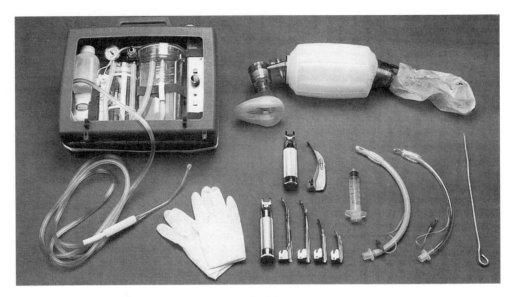

Figure 2-17 Equipment needed for endotracheal intubation.

Equipment (Figure 2-17)

- Laryngoscope blade
- Laryngoscope handle
- ETT
- Syringe (10 cc)
- Stylet
- Water-soluble lubricant
- Suction equipment
- Magill forceps
- Adhesive tape or ETT tube holder
- BVM
- Oxygen
- Gloves
- Goggles

The ETT is a curved plastic tube with a low-pressure cuff near the distal end (Figure 2-18). The tube is open at both ends. The proximal end is fitted with a 15-mm adapter for connection to ventilating devices. The cuff is attached to a one-way valve through a side tube that has a pilot balloon to indicate whether or not the cuff is inflated (Figure 2-19). The tube has various markings (in centimeters) to indicate the distance from the tip. The size of the tube is expressed in terms of its internal diameter (ID).

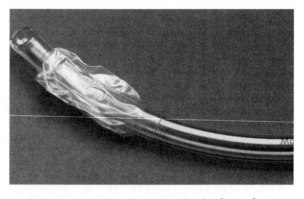

Figure 2-18 The endotracheal tube has a low-pressure cuff near the distal end.

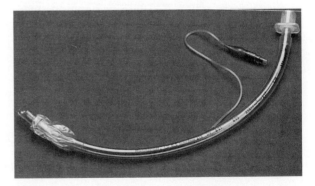

Figure 2-19 The cuff is attached to a one-way valve and pilot balloon.

The laryngoscope blade can be either curved (MacIntosh) or straight (Miller). The choice of which blade to use is a matter of personal preference. Since the curved blade is inserted into the vallecula and lifts the epiglottis indirectly, it is thought by some to be more "physiologic" and less traumatic. In a short, thick-necked individual, the curved blade may facilitate visualization. In children, straight blades are preferred.

Blades come in different sizes. Most adults can be intubated with a No. 3 or No. 4 blade. Infants and children, depending on their age, need No. 0 to No. 2 blades. The blade has a bulb near its distal end. It is important to check and ascertain that the bulb is tightly secured in its socket. Newer models have fiber-optic lights with the light source in the handle; hence there will not be a bulb to tighten.

The laryngoscope handle contains batteries for the light bulb in the blade. The handle has a bar at its top onto which fits the indentation of the blade (Figure 2-20). When fitted properly and snapped into a 90-degree angle, electrical connection is made, and the bulb is turned on (Figure 2-21). When the blade is collapsed to the side of the handle, the light goes off (Figure 2-22).

The stylet is a malleable guide that can be inserted into the ETT. This allows the tube to be shaped in optimal curvature to facilitate intubation, somewhat like the letter J. The stylet should be recessed ½ inch from the distal end of the tube. Once the stylet is inserted, it is advisable to bend the proximal end over the 15-mm adapter of the tube so that it will not accidentally slide down farther. Some stylets are manufactured with a loop at the proximal end to prevent accidental slipping (Figure 2-23). Others are provided with a plastic stopper to prevent them from sliding inadvertently into the tube. The stopper fits into the adapter (Figure 2-24).

The Magill forceps have a long handle that is bent at an obtuse angle in the middle. The tips have rings with serrated inner surfaces to

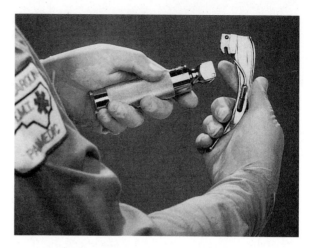
Figure 2-20 Always check to make sure that the bulb is screwed in tight before laryngoscopy.

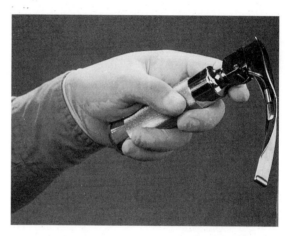
Figure 2-21 When fitted properly, the bulb will light when the blade is in the 90-degree position.

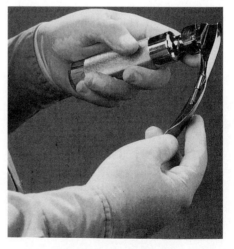
Figure 2-22 When the blade is collapsed to the side, the light goes off.

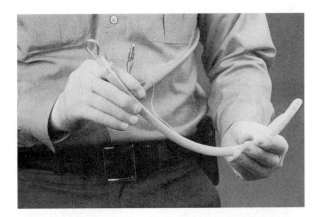

Figure 2-23 Always bend the proximal end of the stylet to prevent accidental tearing of the trachea.

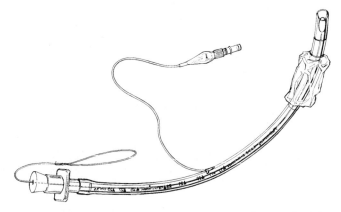

Figure 2-24 Some stylets are manufactured with loops or stoppers near their proximal ends.

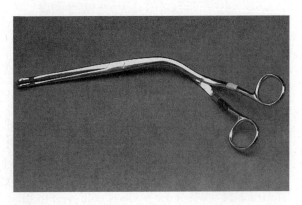

Figure 2-25 Magill Forceps

facilitate grasping. Occasionally these tubes are required to guide the tube into the larynx. Care should be taken not to grasp the balloon with the forceps, since the teeth on the forceps may rupture the balloon (Figure 2-25).

Anatomy of the Upper Airway

Figures 2-26 through 2-29 show the side and the laryngoscopic view of the airway. The pharynx is a fibromuscular tube that extends from the base of the skull to the cricoid cartilage, where it becomes the esophagus. The larynx, situated in front of the pharynx, is mostly composed of cartilages. The thyroid, cricoid, and arytenoid cartilages form the bulk of the larynx (Figure 2-26). In addition, the epiglottis and two each of cuneiform and corniculate cartilages form the upper ring (Figure 2-27). The epiglottis is a cartilaginous fold that protrudes posterior and cephalad (toward the scalp), starting at the base of the tongue. It overhangs the glottic opening, through which the vocal cords can be seen. The vallecula is a small indentation found between the base of the tongue and the epiglottis.

When the laryngoscope blade is inserted into the mouth, the epiglottis comes into view. Beyond the epiglottis the vocal cords are seen. They appear as two folds shaped like an inverted V. The tracheal rings can sometimes be seen through the opening between the vocal cords (Figures 2-28 and 2-29).

The alignment of the three axes of the upper airway is crucial during intubation. The oropharyngeal, the pharyngoglottic, and the glottic tracheal axes can be aligned with the sniffing position by the classic chin-lift/head-tilt or jaw-thrust maneuvers (Figure 2-30).

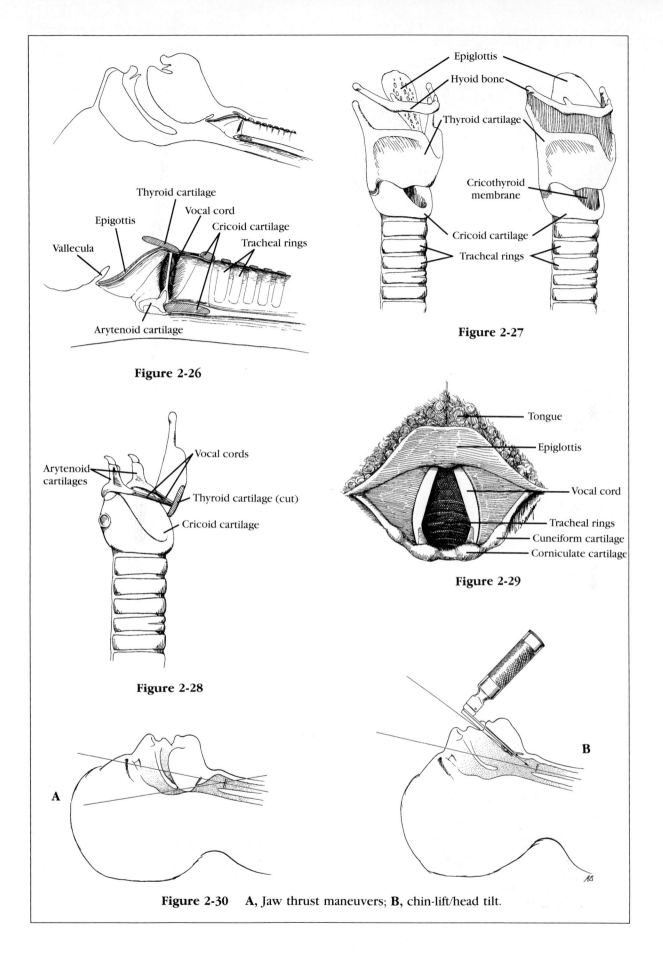

Figure 2-26

Figure 2-27

Figure 2-28

Figure 2-29

Figure 2-30   **A,** Jaw thrust maneuvers; **B,** chin-lift/head tilt.

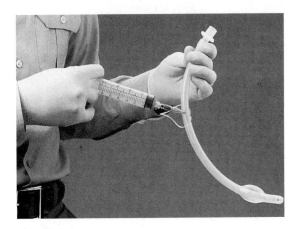

Figure 2-31 Check the cuff for air leaks.

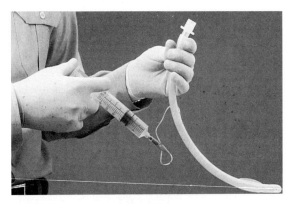

Figure 2-32 Leave the syringe filled with air attached to the one-way valve.

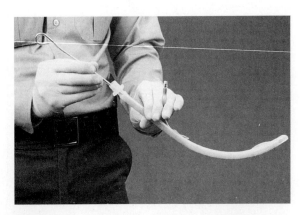

Figure 2-33 Bend the proximal end of the stylet to prevent it from sliding farther down into the tube.

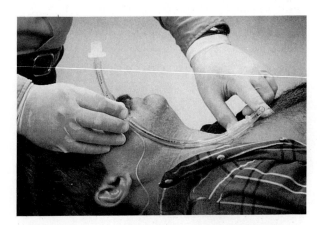

Figure 2-34 Estimate the length of the tube.

Procedure

1. Observe universal precautions.

2. Continue CPR and mask ventilation while preparing to intubate.

3. Set up the suction unit with a rigid tonsil-tip (Yankauer) catheter.

4. Choose the proper size ETT and blade.

5. Assemble the laryngoscope and check the light.

6. Check the ETT cuff for air leaks (Figure 2-31). Open the top of the ETT package and inflate the cuff through the valve with 10 cc of air. Once you are satisfied that there is no leak, deflate the cuff. Leave the syringe filled with air attached to the valve (Figure 2-32). Keep the ETT in its package to ensure sterility.

7. Insert a guide (stylet) into the ETT. Be careful not to push the stylet through the tip of the ETT. Make sure that the stylet is recessed at least ½ inch from the tip. Bend the proximal end of the stylet over the ETT to prevent it from accidentally sliding farther down into the tube (Figure 2-33).

8. Remove the ETT from its package and liberally lubricate the distal 3 or 4 inches and the balloon. You may use water-soluble lubricating jelly or, if permitted in your system, lidocaine jelly or ointment. Estimate the length of the tube needed by placing it alongside the patient's cheek and neck to the level of the cri-

coid cartilage (Figure 2-34). Then replace the ETT in its package.

9. Preoxygenate the patient by bagging with 100% oxygen at the rate of one ventilation per second, for 10 to 15 seconds.

10. Stop ventilations and remove the facemask.

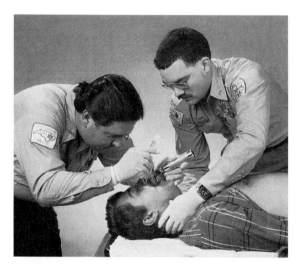

Figure 2-35 In-line stabilization can be held while intubating.

11. Use your right hand to open the mouth.

12. With the head-tilt/chin-lift maneuver, the sniffing position is achieved. This aligns the airway axes. In trauma, or when cervical spine integrity is questioned, **DO NOT** hyperextend the neck. In-line cervical immobilization should be applied by a second rescuer, who places himself or herself by the side of the patient, below the patient's shoulder level, and stabilizes the jaw, neck, and head as shown (Figure 2-35). In this position the rescuer providing cervical spine immobilization will not hinder the intubator's line of vision.

13. While holding the laryngoscope handle in the left hand, insert the blade into the mouth on the right side of the patient, pushing the tongue toward the left. Do not touch the teeth with the blade (Figure 2-36).

14. Under direct vision, insert the blade down to the base of the tongue and visualize the epiglottis (Figure 2-37). A common error is to push the blade down without properly visualizing the epiglottis and then to try to "fish"

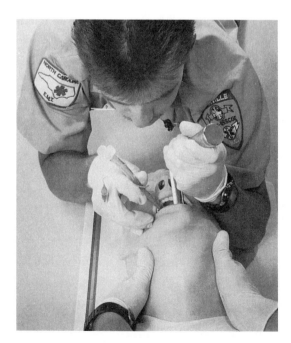

Figure 2-36 Do not touch the teeth with the blade.

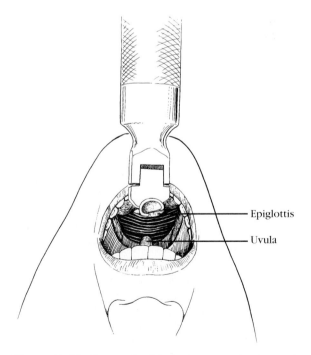

Figure 2-37 Insert the blade down to the base of the tongue and visualize the epiglottis.

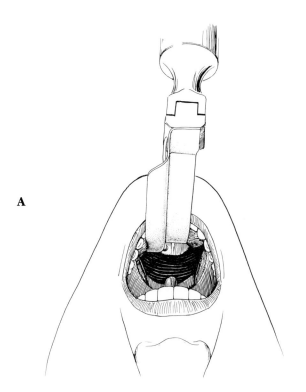

A

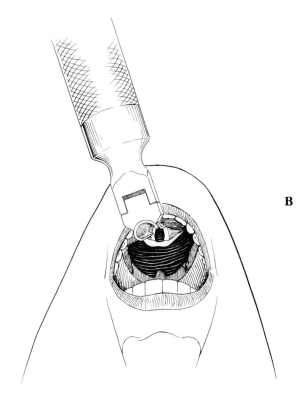

B

Figure 2-38 **A**, The distal tip of the curved blade is placed into the vallecula. **B**, The straight blade lifts the epiglottis to visualize the vocal cords.

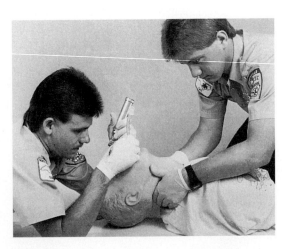

Figure 2-39 The paramedic must be able to see the tube entering the trachea.

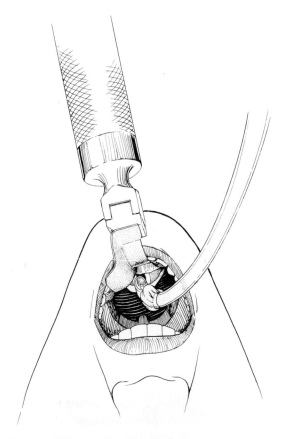

Figure 2-40 The experienced paramedic can often "feel" the cuff pass through the vocal cords.

it out by moving the blade tip with chaotic and random motion. This not only causes trauma, but it also causes the tongue to fall around the blade, occluding landmarks. Use suction as needed. Ideally the intubating time should not be more than 30 seconds. If the intubation is difficult, stop the procedure, hyperventilate the patient with the BVM, and reattempt the procedure.

15. Once you visualize the epiglottis, the next step is to identify the vocal cords. If you are using a curved blade, direct it into the vallecula (between the tongue and the epiglottis) and lift up on the handle and blade (Figure 2-38, *A*). **DO NOT USE THE PATIENT'S TEETH AS A FULCRUM!** If you are using a straight blade, pass it below the epiglottis and lift it up (Figure 2-38, *B*). As you lift the epiglottis by either method, the vocal cords will come into view. Once you can see the vocal cords, try not to take your eyes off of them.

16. Insert the tube into the mouth along the right cheek of the patient. Be careful that your own hand does not obstruct the view of the tube entering through the vocal cords. (Guide the tube from the side of the face.) You must be able to see the tube entering the trachea (Figures 2-39 and 2-40). After you achieve some expertise, you can feel the tube pass through the vocal cords. Beware that the tube has been known to slip down into the esophagus at the last possible moment.

17. Insert the tube until the cuff has entered the trachea completely. Usually, the 22- or 23-cm mark on the tube will be at the patient's incisors. The average distance between the lips to the carina is 28.5 cm in males and 25.2 cm in females. In children the following formula will help in positioning the tube:

Child's age/2 plus 12 = centimeter mark at the teeth

18. Remove the laryngoscope. Secure the tube firmly with your thumb and forefinger. Remove the stylet from the tube. Have your assistant ventilate through the tube, watching for

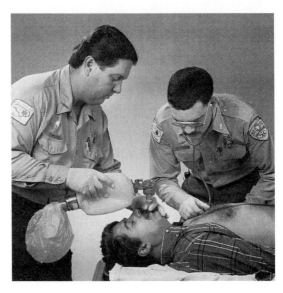

Figure 2-41 Auscultate over both lungs and the epigastric area.

the rising and falling of the chest. Auscultate over both lung fields and the stomach to ensure accurate placement (Figure 2-41).

19. Inflate the cuff until the pilot balloon feels tight and there is no air leak around the balloon (about 7 to 10 cc of air). Remove the syringe.

20. Tape the tube in place securely. This can be achieved by various means. One standard method is to use cloth tape. Select a long piece of tape sufficient to go around the patient's head, with an extra 3 inches to spare at both ends. The adhesive surface of another piece of tape is placed over the adhesive surface of the first tape to prevent the tape from sticking to the patient's hair. The 3-inch lengths of the first tape at both ends should have available adhesive surfaces for wrapping around the tube. These ends are split longitudinally and braided over the tube. Commercially available tube holders may also be used and are much quicker than tape.

21. Recheck breath sounds after any manipulation.

22. Check the pilot balloon periodically to ascertain proper seal and when you suspect air

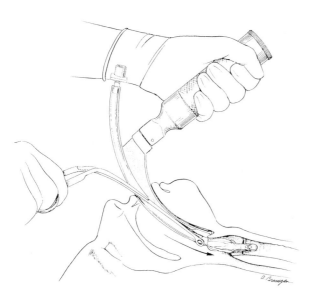

Figure 2-42 Magill forceps can be used to help place the tube into the trachea.

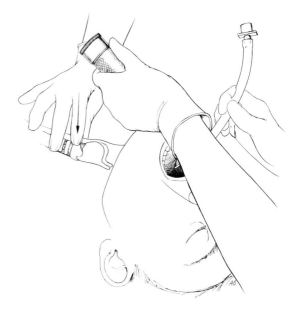

Figure 2-43 Sellick's maneuver is performed by placing gentle pressure on the cricoid ring.

PEARLS
&
PITFALLS

Endotracheal Tips

- A curved blade may provide better visualization in persons with a short, thick neck. A straight blade is often more advantageous in patients with a long, thin neck.
- Sometimes the trachea is positioned more anteriorly than usual. The use of Magill forceps may facilitate intubation by allowing manual guiding of the tube through the vocal cords (Figure 2-42).
- Gentle cricoid pressure by an assistant may help with visualization of the vocal cords (Sellick's maneuver). This maneuver also helps prevent aspiration of gastric contents (Figure 2-43). Do not use this maneuver when the patient is awake because it may in itself induce regurgitation and aspiration.

- Intubation by digitally guiding the tube into the larynx can be useful. This involves inserting two fingers into the mouth, feeling the epiglottis, and manually guiding the tube under the epiglottis. The patient must be unresponsive for this technique to be used successfully. Bite blocks are recommended. There is a danger of the rescuer's fingers getting bitten (see Figure 2-49). This technique is advocated by some EMS systems, but it requires some experience and dexterity. Also, it should be emphasized that this is a blind technique and lacks the advantages of direct visualization discussed earlier.
- Using a lighted stylet to intubate is another technique that may sometimes be useful. When the tube is passed blindly toward the epiglottis, the anterior neck is examined for transillumination. If the tube enters the trachea, the light will be seen in the midline.

leak. Also, if the patient vomits, it is prudent to check the pilot balloon to make sure that there is no danger of aspiration.

Complications of endotracheal intubation

Early
- Tooth damage
- Injury to pharynx, resulting in bleeding, hematoma, or perforation
- Aspiration of a tooth or laryngoscope bulb
- Bronchial intubation
- Cervical fracture, subluxation
- Tracheal perforation
- Pneumothorax
- Subcutaneous and mediastinal emphysema
- Aspiration (around inflated cuff)

- Cardiac dysrhythmias
- Increase in intracranial pressure
- Esophageal intubation

Late
- Overinflated cuff, which may cause necrosis or perforation
- Fistula formation (tracheoesophageal, tracheopleural)
- Stenosis of the trachea
- Synechiae of vocal cords (cords stick together with fibrous tissue, resulting in alteration or loss of voice)
- Vocal cord paralysis

Rapid sequence induction

As noted earlier, emergency intubation poses the potential hazard for increase in in-

Medications for Intubation

It is not often necessary to use medications for intubation in emergency situations. Occasionally an alert individual may have to be intubated. Victims of severe head injuries have been known to develop increase in intracranial pressure following any therapeutic manipulation. Hypoxia, drug abuse, and hypovolemia may cause combativeness.

Some of the common medications used for sedation are:
- Minor tranquilizers such as diazepam (usual dose: 2 to 5 mg intravenously), midazolam (0.05 to 0.1 mg/kg titrated slowly in increments of 1 to 2 mg every 2 minutes).
- Major tranquilizers such as droperidol (2.5 to 5 mg intravenously, titrated to achieve desired effect), haloperidol (2 to 5 mg intravenously, titrated)
- Narcotics such as morphine sulphate (titrated in increments of 2 to 3 mg intravenously to a maximum of 10 to 15 mg intravenously), fentanyl (1 to 2 µg/kg intravenously; average adult dose 0.025 to 0.05 mg intravenously). The effects of these two drugs can be reversed with naloxone.

In addition to the sedatives, certain muscle relaxants can be used to induce skeletal muscle paralysis. These include depolarizing agents such as succinylcholine chloride (Sch) and nondepolarizing agents such as pancuronium and norcuronium. The use of muscle relaxants during emergency intubation is hazardous. They should only be used by personnel who are thoroughly familiar with their use.

SCh causes brief muscle fasciculations followed by paralysis within 60 seconds. The action lasts only for about 5 to 10 minutes. Because of its rapidity of action, SCh is the preferred agent for intubation in emergencies. However, the fasciculations can lead to hyperkalemia, myoglobinemia, and myoglobinuria. Contractions of the abdominal muscles may lead to regurgitation of gastric contents. Pancuronium and other nondepolarizing agents are slow to induce paralysis, and their action lasts for about an hour. This makes them less desirable in emergency situations. Because of their longer duration of action, these agents are more suitable for maintaining paralysis **after** intubation.

tracranial pressure and cardiac dysrhythmias. When possible, follow the procedure outlined here to help protect the patient.

Preoxygenate the patient with 100% oxygen. This offers protection against subsequent hypoxia. Make sure all necessary supplies and medications are available. Keep a cricothyrotomy tray ready. If possible, have a crew member assist you with the setup. The patient may be sedated at this point, using either morphine sulphate, fentanyl, diazepam, or midazolam (check with local protocols). Have the assistant perform the Sellick maneuver. Some authorities prefer to give a priming dose of pancuronium at this time (0.01 mg/kg intravenously), to prevent fasciculations that will later develop from the use of succinylcholine (SCh). After the pancuronium, administer lidocaine (1 mg/kg intravenously). This blunts the rise in intracranial pressure. General anesthesia is induced using thiopental sodium (3 to 4 mg/kg). In prehospital situations, fentanyl or morphine sulphate titrated to cause deep sedation may suffice. This is followed by SCh (1 to 2 mg/kg). Intubation is carried out orotracheally. After the tube is secured in place, additional sedatives or paralytic agents may be administered.

♦ Nasotracheal Intubation

Background

Although the concept and technique of nasotracheal intubation were developed during World War I, the procedure was used only occasionally in the operating suite. Recently, however, emergency physicians and paramedics have sparked a renewed interest in the procedure.

Indications

Any person who is in need of intubation but has spontaneous respirations can be intubated nasotracheally (e.g., drug overdose, head injury, COPD, congestive heart failure, pneumonia, and asthma).

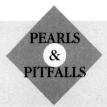

Advantages and Disadvantages of Nasotracheal Intubation

Advantages

- It can be used on patients with injury to the cervical spine, since the risk of movement is minimal compared to orotracheal intubation.
- Awake patients tolerate a tube through the nose better than one through the mouth.
- Sometimes it is difficult to open a patient's mouth. Trismus (spasm of the jaw) can be caused by closed head injury, decerebrate rigidity, seizures, facial injuries, and certain infections.

Disadvantages

- Nasotracheal intubation is a blind procedure. It should not be used in cases of suspected foreign body airway obstruction.
- It may cause excessive bleeding from the nose or posterior pharyngeal area.
- In the presence of basilar skull fracture, a tube inserted blindly through the nose may perforate the base of the skull and enter the brain tissue (Figure 2-44).
- The patient should be breathing spontaneously. Therefore, this technique cannot be used in cases of cardiopulmonary arrest for which intubation is commonly performed in prehospital care.

Contraindications

- Apnea
- Airway obstruction caused by foreign bodies
- Severe facial injury/basilar skull fracture
- Bleeding disorders

NOTE: There is an increased risk of infections such as meningitis associated with this procedure, especially in people with cardiac valve problems or prosthesis. Therefore it is relatively contraindicated in these patients.

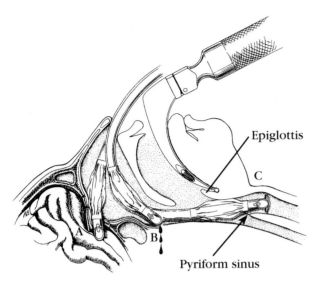

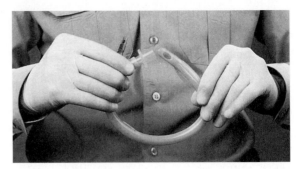

Figure 2-45 Forming a circle with an ETT will help you ensure a curvature when performing nasal intubation.

Figure 2-44 This diagram shows three complications of nasotracheal intubation: *A*, Tube entering the cranial cavity; *B*, tube causing bleeding in the nasopharynx; and *C*, tube damaging the vocal cords.

Equipment

- ETT (7 to 8 ID for most adults)
- 10-cc syringe
- Lidocaine jelly (or water-soluble)
- Topical anesthetic spray (e.g., benzocaine)
- Laryngoscope with a No. 3 curved blade
- Magill forceps
- Tape
- Gloves
- Goggles
- BVM
- Oxygen
- Suction equipment

Procedure

1. Observe universal precautions.

2. Select an ETT (usually 7.5 mm ID in males, 7 mm ID in females). It is usually 0.5 mm smaller than the tube that would be used if orotracheal intubation were going to be performed. Check the cuff. Lubricate the tube with lidocaine jelly. Insert the distal end of the ETT into its proximal adapter to form a circle and set it aside (Figure 2-45). This ensures slight anterior curvature of the tube to facilitate en-

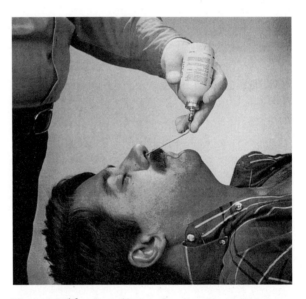

Figure 2-46 Anesthetize the nostrils and pharynx if time permits.

try into the trachea. No stylet is used in this procedure.

3. Anesthetize the nostrils and pharynx. Benzocaine topical anesthetic spray can be used for this purpose (Figure 2-46). Lidocaine spray (2%) can also be used. Usually, in the prehospital setting, there is no time for adequate topical anesthesia. You can use a vasoconstrictor spray such as phenylephrine hydrochloride ½% or 1% to shrink the mucous membranes. You can place a nasopharyngeal airway before you attempt to keep the nasal passage open. Have suction equipment available at all times.

4. Pick up the tube and release the circle previously formed. Taking care not to straighten the tip of the tube, insert it through either the right or the left nostril. Keep the bevel of the tube toward the septum.

5. Gently insert the tube until the tip is in the nasopharynx. Continue to push the tube down. Listen and look for breath sounds and vapor condensation through the tube (Figure 2-47, *A* and *B*).

6. As the tube approaches the larynx, the sounds of breathing through the tube get louder. Gently and evenly push the tube into the larynx during inspiration.

7. The 15-mm adapter usually rests close to the nostril. On entering the trachea, the tube may stimulate the gag reflex and make the patient cough and buck. Be prepared to control the cervical spine. Watch for vomiting.

8. If the tube enters the esophagus, the patient may moan. Ventilate the patient and auscultate over both lungs and the epigastrium. If the tube is found to be in the esophagus, withdraw it until the tip is in the pharynx and try

again. Pushing the tube down during the patient's inspiratory efforts will greatly enhance your chances for a successful intubation.

There is no need to jab the tube unduly and forcibly through the vocal cords, "hoping to get it in quickly." Force causes violent retching and bucking. Remember that you don't know where the tip of the tube is. You might perforate the pyriform sinus, lacerate the epiglottis, shear off the vocal cords, enter the mediastinum, or puncture major blood vessels.

Complications
- Bleeding from the nose
- Retropharyngeal perforation, hematoma
- Nasal septal tear
- Cranial perforation in basilar skull fracture
- Infection such as meningitis, encephalitis, pharyngeal abscess, or endocarditis
- Injury to the pyriform sinus, epiglottis, vocal cords
- Subglottic stenosis
- Complications that accompany insertion of orotracheal tubes

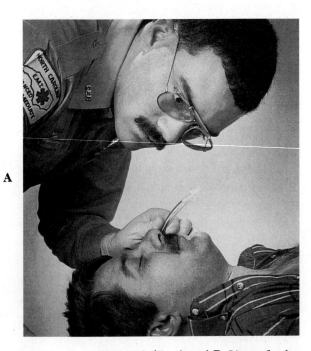
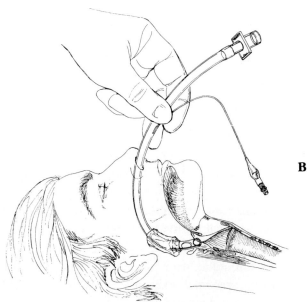

A

B

Figure 2-47 **A** and **B**, Listen for breath sounds and look for vapor in the tube.

PEARLS
&
PITFALLS

If at First You Don't Succeed...

Most people report a 90% success rate with nasotracheal intubation. However, if two or three attempts fail, you may try the following:

• Withdraw the tube and try again through the other nostril. Occasionally you get a better angle from the other side.

• Make sure that the cervical spine is immobilized. Insert a laryngoscope with a curved blade into the mouth. Visualize the vocal cords and the tip of the ETT in the pharynx. Sometimes the tube can be guided into the trachea under direct vision. Frequently, however, you need Magill forceps to direct the tube into the glottic opening (Figure 2-48). Grasp the tube gently with the forceps. Do not pull the tube toward the vocal cords. Have your assistant gently push it through the nose while you guide the tip into the glottis. Remember, the teeth on Magill forceps may damage the balloon on the tube.

• Occasionally, the tube can be guided into the glottic opening by digital manipulation. You should only attempt this if the patient is comatose and therefore unable to bite your fingers. If you are on the right side of the patient, insert your right index and middle fingers into the patient's mouth. Feel the epiglottis and the tube. Gently guide the tube between your fingers under the epiglottis, as you push the proximal end toward the nostril with your other hand (Figure 2-49).

• A ringed ETT (Endotrol) is available. A ring at the proximal end of the tube controls the tip of the tube. By pulling on the ring, the tip can be flexed anteriorly. This essentially replaces forming a circle with the tube described earlier.

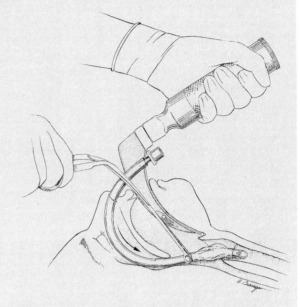

Figure 2-48 Grasp the tube with McGill forceps and guide it into the trachea.

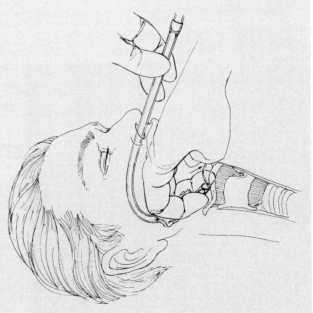

Figure 2-49 Guide the end of the tube with your fingers.

Anatomy for the Cricothyrotomy

The EMS provider should become familiar with the anatomic landmarks of the neck. If you run your finger down the midline beginning at the chin (mentum), you will come across a cartilaginous mound that has a V-shaped notch superiorly. This is the thyroid cartilage (Adam's apple). As you move your finger about 2 to 3 cm farther down, you will feel a flat space, followed by another cartilage. This second bump is the cricoid cartilage. The space between these two cartilages is covered by the cricothyroid membrane. In the adult this membrane measures 9 mm vertically and 3 cm horizontally (Figure 2-50, *A* and *B*). A small artery traverses the membrane in its superior aspect. If you continue to move your finger down the midline, you will feel the tracheal rings in the suprasternal notch.

◆ Surgical Cricothyrotomy (Cricothyroidotomy)

Background

It is said that the first tracheostomy was performed by the Greek physician, Asclepiades. In the late nineteenth century, surgeons started performing cricothyrotomy because of ease of performance. The technique was not standardized. The incision was made anywhere in the anterior neck. In 1909, Dr. Chevalier Jackson, a prominent surgeon and a pioneer of his time, standardized the technique of tracheotomy. Dr. Jackson saw so many complications occur following cricothyrotomy performed by his colleagues that in 1921 he utterly condemned "high tracheotomy," as he called it.

Because of Dr. Jackson's influence in the world of medicine, cricothyrotomy became an almost extinct procedure until the 1960s. At that time, because of advances in medicine, the availability of antibiotics, and the changing pattern of disease processes, numerous investigators began "revisiting" cricothyrotomy.

Although complications can and do occur, if tracheal intubation cannot be performed, cricothyrotomy is the next obvious choice.

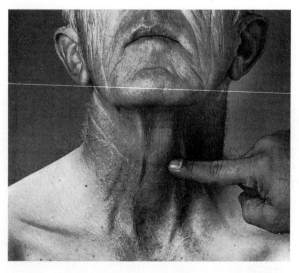
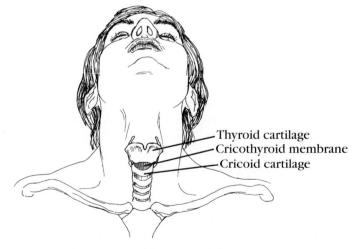

Thyroid cartilage
Cricothyroid membrane
Cricoid cartilage

Figure 2-50 **A** and **B**, The cricothyroid membrane is found between the thyroid cartilage (Adam's apple) and the cricoid cartilage.

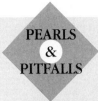

Advantages and Disadvantages of Cricothyrotomy

Advantages

* It is faster than a tracheostomy.
* Surgical skill required can be taught to nonsurgeons easily.
* It **can** be done in the field.
* Since the cricoid cartilage is shaped like a ring and encircles the larynx, it is difficult for an overzealous operator with a scalpel to damage the esophagus and other posterior structures. On the other hand, the tracheal rings are open posteriorly.
* It can be performed without movement of the cervical spine.

Disadvantages

* It can potentially result in subglottic stenosis (stricture of the larynx below the glottis).
* Even though no major surgical skill is required to perform cricothyrotomy, it should be remembered that it **is** an invasive procedure and knowledge of the anatomy and familiarization with the procedure are necessary.
* Swelling of the anterior neck may mask landmarks.

Indications

It should be emphasized that the only indication for cricothyrotomy is the inability to secure an airway by other noninvasive procedures such as endotracheal intubation (e.g., cervical spine trauma, maxillofacial trauma, oropharyngeal obstruction caused by foreign body, masses, infections (epiglottitis), edema resulting from allergic reactions, or inhalation injury.

Contraindications

* Possibility of establishing an easier and less invasive airway rapidly
* Acute laryngeal disorders such as laryngeal fractures that cause distortion or obliteration of landmarks (e.g., children under 10 years of age, bleeding disorders, injury or obstruction below the level of the cricothyroid membrane)

Equipment (Figure 2-51)

* A sterile fenestrated drape (hole in the center)
* Prepared antiseptic swab sticks such as povidone-iodine
* Scalpel with a No. 11 or a No. 15 blade
* 4×4 gauze pads
* ETT (7.5 mm ID), or Shiley tracheostomy tube (No. 4 or No. 5), cuffed; the ETT should be shortened to about 3 inches, in-

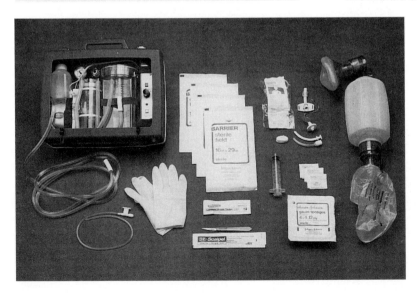

Figure 2-51 Equipment necessary to perform a cricothyrotomy.

cluding the cuff and the pilot balloon; the 15-mm adapter is removed from the proximal end and fitted into the cut edge of the distal end; the proximal portion of the tube is discarded

• 10-cc syringe to inflate the cuff
• Two arterial clamps (hemostats)—8-inch and 6-inch
• Sterile gloves
• Suction equipment
• BVM
• Oxygen
• Adhesive or umbilical cord tape
• Goggles

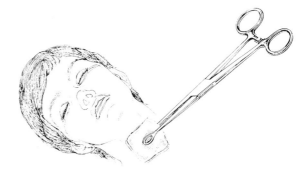

Figure 2-52 Prep the neck with povidone-iodine.

Procedure

1. Observe universal precautions. Put on sterile gloves.

2. The patient should be in a supine position. Immobilize the neck if necessary.

3. Open the cricothyrotomy kit.

4. Make sure that artificial ventilation is in progress by means of a BVM while preparing for the procedure.

5. Prepare povidone-iodine swab sticks.

6. Surgically prepare the entire anterior neck (Figure 2-52).

7. Drape the area with the fenestrated sheet.

8. Palpate the thyroid notch, cricothyroid membrane, and the sternal notch; orient yourself thoroughly with the landmarks (Figure 2-53).

9. Stabilize the thyroid cartilage with your left hand (or nondominant hand). This is the most important step. If you lose the midline, the anatomy will be distorted and you may find yourself in muscles and blood vessels on either side.

10. Make a transverse (horizontal) skin incision over the cricothyroid membrane, over its lower half. Try to cut through the skin and the subcutaneous tissue in one clean, bold stroke. Make this incision at least 2 cm long (Figure 2-54).

11. There will be some brisk bleeding. Sponge it if necessary, but don't waste too much time trying to stop it.

12. With your index finger, feel the cricothy-

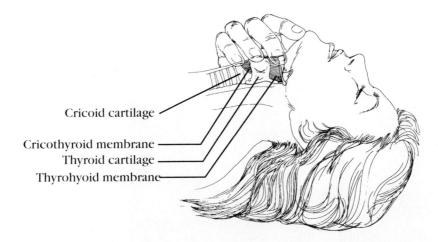

Cricoid cartilage
Cricothyroid membrane
Thyroid cartilage
Thyrohyoid membrane

Figure 2-53 Orient yourself thoroughly with the landmarks of the neck.

roid membrane. Carefully make a horizontal incision over the lower part of the membrane.

13. Insert the scalpel handle into the incision and rotate it 90 degrees to open the airway (Figure 2-55). If the patient is breathing spontaneously, secretions, blood, and air will spray out of the opening. **Protect your face.**

14. Insert the tracheostomy tube (Figure 2-56, *A* and *B*) into the opening. A shortened ETT (with the cuff and the pilot balloon intact) can be used in lieu of the tracheostomy tube.

15. Inflate the cuff and ventilate the patient.

16. Observe the chest rise and fall; auscultate the lungs and the stomach to ensure proper tube placement.

17. Secure the tube to the patient by adhesive tape or umbilical cord tape.

Complications

* Bleeding
* Infection; cellulitis, tracheitis, pneumonia
* False passage creation resulting in pneumomediastinum, pneumothorax
* Subglottic stenosis
* Tracheal or esophageal injury

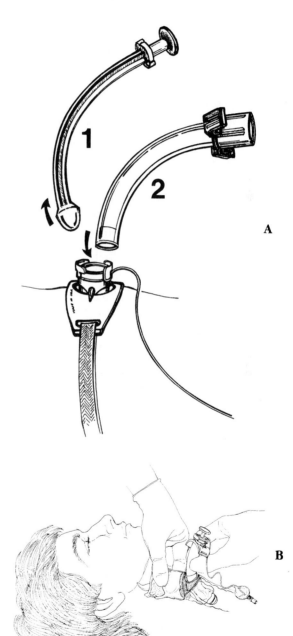

A

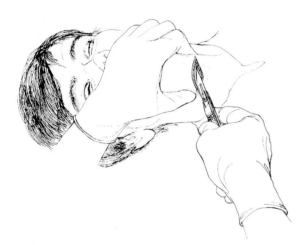

Figure 2-54 Stabilize the thyroid cartilage while making a 2-cm incision.

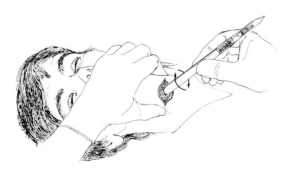

Figure 2-55 Insert the scalpel handle and rotate it 90 degrees.

B

Figure 2-56 **A** and **B**, Secure the tracheostomy tube holder with the provided tie. Remove the obturator *(1)* and insert the tracheostomy tube *(2)*.

• Fistula formation
• Tube dislodgement
• Mucus plug
• Apnea, cardiac arrest

In addition to the technique described in the preceding paragraphs, other methods have been described. Some advocate the use of a vertical incision on the skin (followed by a transverse incision on the cricothyroid membrane). The obvious advantage is that, if the incision is made inadvertently at a wrong level, it can be extended up or down. Also, the risk of cutting through the lateral structures (strap muscles of the neck and the blood vessels) is minimized. Commercially available instruments have also been used. These are called "cricothyrotomes." The Nu-Trake is an example of such a device that has a trocar and a sheath. The instrument is pushed through the cricothyroid membrane, the trocar is removed, and the sheath inserted into the larynx. Care should be taken not to push the trocar through the posterior wall or the cricoid cartilage.

◆ Percutaneous Transtracheal Ventilation (Needle Cricothyrotomy)

Background

In situations in which endotracheal intubation is not possible, cricothyrotomy continues to be the next choice. Cricothyrotomy is a surgical procedure and requires training before it can be performed. Percutaneous transtracheal ventilation (PTV) is a viable alternative to surgical cricothyrotomy and may be more suitable in the prehospital scene.

PTV involves the insertion of a catheter through the cricothyroid membrane. The catheter is then connected to a high-pressure oxygen source, and oxygen is delivered intermittently into the trachea. The trepidation that accompanies performing a surgical procedure such as cricothyrotomy makes PTV an attractive alternative. The procedure can be accom-

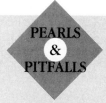

PEARLS & PITFALLS

Caution

• PTV is an invasive procedure and requires proper training and certification. It should only be done with the approval of your EMS system.
• Even though it sounds simple, carbon dioxide (CO_2) buildup occurs rapidly; hence the procedure can be used only for a short period of time (30 minutes). A definitive airway such as surgical cricothyrotomy must still be established.

plished in a short time and may be used before performing cricothyrotomy.

Indications

• The only indication for cricothyrotomy is the inability to secure an airway by other noninvasive procedures such as endotracheal intubation (e.g., cervical spine trauma; maxillofacial trauma; and oropharyngeal obstruction caused by foreign body, masses, infections (epiglottitis), or edema resulting from allergic reactions or inhalation injury)

Contraindications

• Possibility of establishing an easier and less invasive airway rapidly
• Acute laryngeal disorders such as laryngeal fractures that cause distortion or obliteration of landmarks (e.g., children under 10 years of age, bleeding disorders, injury or obstruction below the level of the cricothyroid membrane)

Equipment (Figure 2-57)

• 14-gauge or larger over-the-needle catheter, 2¼ inches long

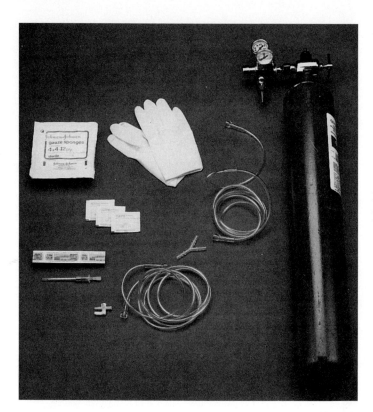

Figure 2-57 Equipment needed for performing percutaneous transtracheal ventilation.

- 10-cc syringe
- Three-way stopcock
- Two standard oxygen tubings, 4 to 5 feet each
- Y-connector
- Oxygen cylinder coupled with 50-psi step-down regulator and needle flow meter (e.g., Bourdon-type flow gauge and regulator)
- Povidone-iodine swabs
- Adhesive tape
- Suction equipment
- Gloves
- Goggles

Procedure

1. Observe universal precautions.

2. Palpate the thyroid cartilage, cricothyroid membrane, and suprasternal notch.

3. Prep the skin with two povidone-iodine swabs.

4. You may attach the syringe to the over-the-needle catheter, or you may elect to use the catheter-needle assembly by itself. Figure 2-58, *A* and *B* shows the use of only a needle and the catheter. This is a personal preference—some think that using a syringe makes the unit less stable. Some may argue that entry into the larynx is more readily verified with gentle suction using the syringe assembly and that this advantage somewhat outweighs the instability of the unit. Puncture the skin over the cricothyroid membrane (Figure 2-58, *A* and *B*).

5. Advance the needle at a 45-degree angle caudally (toward the feet) (Figure 2-59).

6. Carefully push the needle until it "pops" into the trachea (aspirating on the syringe as you advance the needle, if you are using a syringe).

7. Free movement of air confirms that you are in the trachea.

8. Advance the plastic catheter over the needle, holding the needle stationary, until the catheter hub comes to rest against the skin (Figures 2-60 and 2-61).

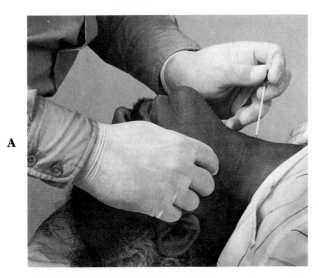

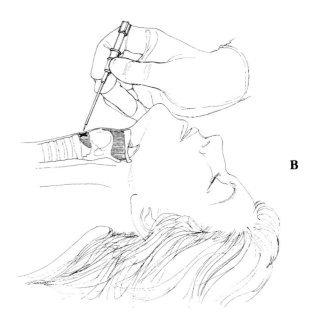

Figure 2-58   **A** and **B**, Puncture the skin over the cricothyroid membrane.

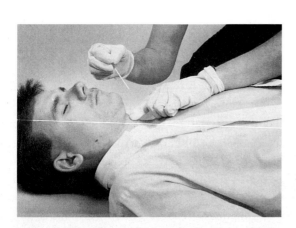

Figure 2-59   Advance the needle at a 45-degree angle caudally.

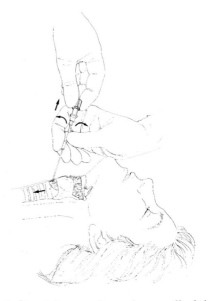

Figure 2-60   Advance the catheter off of the needle into the trachea.

9. Holding the catheter securely, remove the needle.

10. Reconfirm the position of the catheter. Securely tape the catheter to the skin.

11. Attach the three-way stopcock to the catheter hub. Connect one end of the oxygen tubing to the stopcock (Figure 2-62).

12. Connect the other end of the oxygen tubing to the Y-connector. Attach the second oxygen tubing to the other arm of the Y-connector. This tubing is then connected to the flowmeter on the oxygen cylinder. These

connections should be made before the procedure to save time (Figure 2-63).

13. To ventilate the patient, open the regulator and set it at maximum rate (greater than 15 L/min). Occlude the third arm of the Y-connector with your thumb. Air will then flow into the lungs. When you release the occlusion on the Y-connector, air flow will be di-

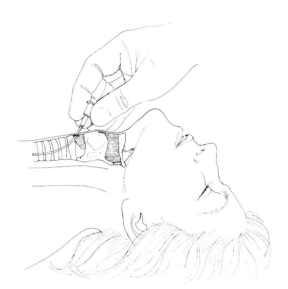

Figure 2-61   Stabilize the catheter.

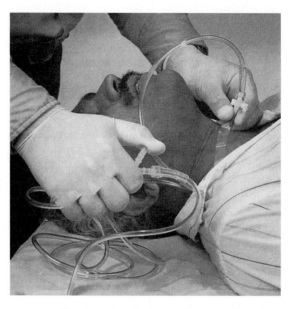

Figure 2-62   Attach a three-way stopcock and oxygen tubing to the catheter.

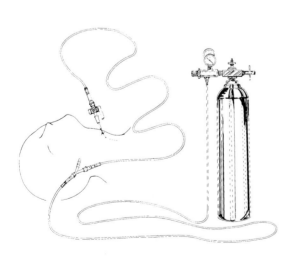

Figure 2-63   Ventilation devices such as this can be prepared before you need them in the field.

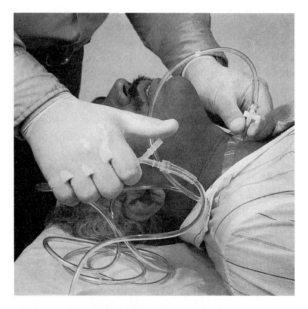

Figure 2-64   Alternately occlude and release pressure on the connector to ventilate the patient, using a 1:4 ratio.

verted outward, allowing the lungs to recoil and collapse (Figure 2-64). By alternately occluding and releasing thumb pressure on the connector (1 second on and 4 seconds off), you can maintain adequate ventilation for approximately 30 minutes.

14. Constantly monitor the patient's breath sounds, ventilation status and color. Adequate exhalation never fully occurs with this technique. The patient may develop hypercarbia (increased CO_2) and increased air pressure in the lungs, possibly causing the alveoli to rupture.

Complications

- Pneumothorax
- Pneumomediastinum
- Subcutaneous emphysema
- Catheter dislodgement
- Hemorrhage
- Esophageal or mediastinal injury
- Hypercarbia

◆ Suctioning the Patient

Background

Suctioning the mouth and pharynx may be necessary to clear secretions to visualize the field before intubation.

In addition, when secretions interfere with BVM ventilation or when the patient is unable to clear secretions, aggressive suctioning may be required by the prehospital provider.

While performing direct laryngoscopy or while clearing secretions from the throat during BVM, a rigid tonsil suction device (Yankauer) should be used. Some tonsil suction catheters are equipped with a side thumb port. When the port is occluded, suction is engaged. When the port is released, air is sucked in through the side port and the suction is disengaged. In tonsil suction catheters without the side port, the suction tubing must be crimped to disengage suction.

PEARLS & PITFALLS

More Than One Way...

Numerous alternative methods to achieve ventilation through a needle hole in the cricothyroid membrane have been described. The connections can be made as follows: the adapter from a No. 12 suction catheter (the catheter itself is cut off) fits the hub of the over-the-needle catheter quite well. The oxygen tubing is then attached to this adapter. This eliminates the use of a three-way stopcock.

Using a BVM unit connected to an oxygen source has also been described. Insertion of the catheter into the cricothyroid membrane is performed as described above. The adapter from a 3.5-mm ETT fits on to the hub of the 14-gauge catheter. The ventilating bag is fitted to the adapter in the usual manner (Figure 2-65). Caution should be exercised to ensure adequate exhalation of air. Even though this technique sounds simple, in practice ventilation through a small catheter is quite difficult.

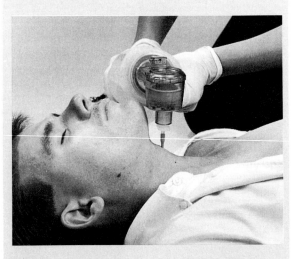

Figure 2-65 A 3.5-mm ETT adapter will fit into the catheter and allow you to ventilate the patient with a BVM.

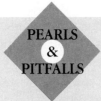

Precautions

During suctioning, oxygen is removed from the tracheobronchial tree. In a patient with an existing relative hypoxia, this may induce cardiac dysrhythmias, apnea, or cardiac arrest. Vigorous suctioning may cause the patient to buck. If cervical spine control is necessary, this may pose a problem.

Always preoxygenate the patient for at least 2 minutes before suctioning if possible. Do not use suction for more than 10 seconds orally or 5 seconds endotracheally at a time. Count "one 1000, two 1000......" from the time you engage the suction.

The tonsil suction must always be used under direct vision. It should not be forced blindly into the patient's mouth because it may push an obstructing foreign body farther into the throat or cause tissue damage and bleeding.

Tracheal Suctioning

Paramedics are called on to perform deep suctioning in many situations—both medical and trauma. When the patient is unable to clear secretions because of illness, overproduction, or very tenacious secretions, airway assistance may be required. In addition, suctioning is commonly done in intubated medical and trauma patients.

Equipment

- Sterile tracheal suctioning kits are available, containing one glove (some kits contain a pair of gloves), a paper cup for sterile saline or water, a suctioning catheter with a side thumb port, a suction unit, goggles, and sterile saline or water.

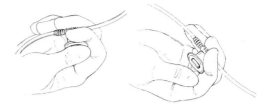

Figure 2-66 Occlude and release the side port with your thumb.

Procedure

1. Observe universal precautions.

2. When you open the kit you will see the sterile glove on top. Put this on your dominant hand, taking care not to touch the outside of the glove with your other hand.

3. Grasp the catheter with the gloved hand. Keep the catheter looped around your hand.

4. With your ungloved hand pour sterile saline solution into the cup provided.

5. Connect the catheter to the suction machine, taking precaution not to touch any other part of the catheter except the proximal tip with your ungloved hand.

6. With the catheter looped around your gloved hand, you should be able to occlude and release the side port with your thumb (Figure 2-66).

7. Feed the catheter through the patient's nose or the ETT (Figure 2-67). It is suggested to use a sterile catheter with each suction attempt. If there are two gloves, you will need an assistant to give you the sterile saline; or you may pour the saline solution into the cup provided before putting on the second glove. This makes it easier to observe absolute sterile precautions.

Procedure for tracheal suctioning the nonintubated patient

1. Place the patient in a semi-sitting position. Unconscious patients are positioned on their side.

2. Supply 100% oxygen for at least 3 minutes.

3. Open the catheter kit and prepare for suctioning.

4. Insert the catheter through a nostril into the pharynx, without engaging the suction (see Figure 2-67).

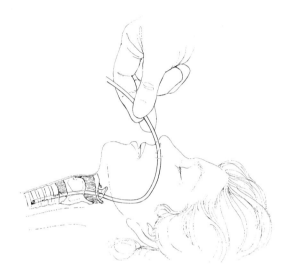

Figure 2-67 Insert the catheter through the patient's nose or ETT.

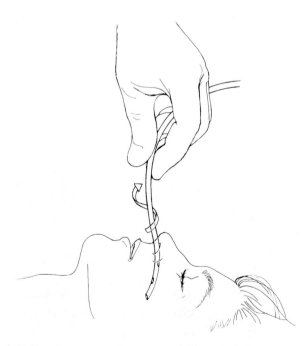

Figure 2-68 Withdraw the catheter using a rotating method.

5. Ask the patient to assume the sniffing position and take slow, deep breaths.

6. Advance the catheter during inspiration. Entering the larynx should induce coughing. Advance through the vocal cords.

7. Engage suction intermittently and withdraw the catheter with a rotating motion (Figure 2-68). Count to 5 seconds or less as needed.

8. When tracheal suctioning is completed, you may use the catheter to suction around the mouth. Once you have suctioned around the mouth, do not introduce the catheter into the trachea again.

9. If you need to use tracheal suctioning again, preoxygenate the patient and repeat the steps, using a new sterile catheter.

10. Dispose of contaminated materials properly.

Procedure for tracheal suctioning of the intubated patient

1. Make sure the patient's cardiac rhythm is being monitored.

2. Preoxygenate with 100% oxygen.

3. Prepare for suctioning. Have an assistant disconnect the bag.

4. Introduce the catheter through the tube without touching the outside of the tube.

5. Advance the catheter as far as possible.

6. Engage intermittent suction and slowly withdraw the catheter. Do not apply suction for more than 5 seconds.

7. Monitor the patient closely. Remember to preoxygenate if you need to suction the patient again. Discontinue suctioning if you see cardiac dysrhythmias, and ventilate the patient with 100% oxygen.

◆ Direct Laryngoscopy for Foreign Body Airway Obstruction

Background

In the event of foreign body airway obstruction (FBAO), subdiaphragmatic abdominal thrusts (Figure 2-69) and finger sweeps should be used to dislodge the foreign body. If these attempts fail, a paramedic may be required to perform direct laryngoscopy and Magill forceps removal of the foreign body.

Procedure

1. Observe universal precautions.

2. Have an assistant attempt BVM ventilation with 100% oxygen.

3. Proceed quickly to direct laryngoscopy.

4. Have tonsil suction and Magill forceps ready.

5. With head tilt/chin lift, bring the patient to the sniffing position and introduce the laryngoscope into the mouth. Insert the blade on the right side of the patient's mouth and push the tongue to the left.

6. Suction if needed. Drop the suction tip and grasp the Magill forceps with your right

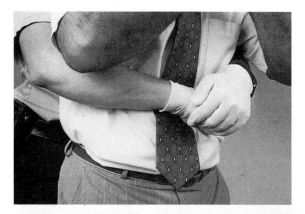

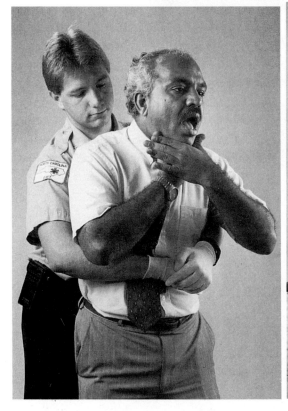
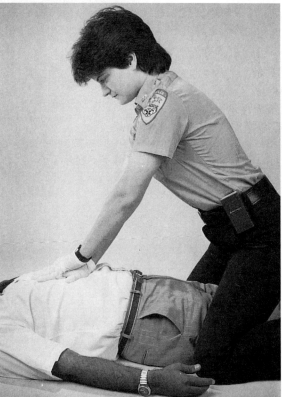

Figure 2-69   Subdiaphragmatic abdominal thrusts are performed.

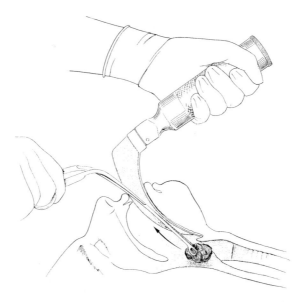

Figure 2-70 Use direct laryngoscopy to visualize the upper airway and remove the foreign body with McGill forceps.

hand. Retrieve the foreign body quickly (Figure 2-70).

7. Immediately withdraw the laryngoscope and attempt to ventilate the patient again, holding proper head position.

8. If you are not able to ventilate, there may be additional foreign bodies. Try direct laryngoscopy again. Repeat abdominal thrusts and direct laryngoscopy until the foreign body is removed. Consider needle cricothyrotomy (percutaneous transtracheal ventilation) or cricothyrotomy if all attempts fail.

◆ Putting It All Together

This chapter has given the prehospital provider many options for managing the patient's airway. However, it must be remembered that all of the advanced devices mean absolutely nothing if he or she fails to open and clear the airway using basic skills. A properly performed jaw-thrust or chin-lift maneuver is still a precursor to all technology. Once the basics have been successfully accomplished and oxygenation established, the advanced tools will provide for improved patient care.

Testing Your Knowledge

1. The cartilaginous fold that protrudes backward and cephalad, starting at the base of the tongue, which prevents aspiration into the trachea, is called the:

   a. Uvula

   b. Epiglottis

   c. Vallecula

   d. Cuneiform cartilage

2. The alignment of three axes of the upper airway is crucial during intubation. Name the three axes.

3. When suctioning a patient orally, the paramedic should suction no longer than seconds. Similarly, tracheal suctioning should last no longer than _____ seconds.

   a. 10,5

   b. 10,10

   c. 5,10

   d. 5,5

4. The purpose of direct laryngoscopy is to allow the paramedic to visualize the:

   a. Epiglottis, trachea, and vocal cords in order to intubate.

   b. Upper airway in order to remove foreign objects obstructing the patient's airway.

   c. Opening of the esophagus in order to place a gastric suction tube.

   d. a and b

5. Endotracheal intubation should be accomplished within what time period?

   a. 30 seconds

   b. 45 seconds

   c. 60 seconds

   d. 90 seconds

6. From the following patients, select the patient in whom the insertion of an EOA would be indicated.

   a. A semi-responsive drug overdose victim

   b. A 60 year-old cardiac arrest of a street person with probable chronic alcohol abuse

   c. A 14-year-old drowning victim

   d. A 56-year-old nonresponsive female whom you are having difficulty intubating with an ETT

7. The EGTA tube is exactly like that of the EOA, except that the EGTA tube has an open lumen on both ends.

   a. True

   b. False

8. The PTL and the ETC are both designed for blind insertion, allowing the operator to place the tube successfully in either the trachea or esophagus.

   a. True

   b. False

9. From the following medications, select the one that is not considered a skeletal muscle relaxant.

   a. Succinylcholine

   b. Pancuronium

   c. Haloperidol

   d. Norcuronium

10. List three contraindications for performing nasotracheal intubation on a patient.

11. The only indication for prehospital cricothyrotomy is the inability to secure an airway by other noninvasive procedures.

    a. True

    b. False

12. Percutaneous transtracheal ventilation is also known as:

    a. Surgical cricothyrotomy.

    b. Digital intubation.

    c. Needle cricothyrotomy.

    d. Tracheal puncture.

Answers are in Appendix A.

BIBLIOGRAPHY

Ampel L: An approach to airway management in the acutely head injured patient, *J Emerg Med* 6:1, 1988.

Asensio JA, Barton JM, Wonsetler LA, et al: Trauma: a systematic approach to management, *Am Fam Physician* 38(3):97-112,1988.

Auerbach PS, Geehr EC: Inadequate oxygenation and ventilation using the EGTA in the prehospital setting, *JAMA* 250:3067, 1983.

Bartlett RL: The pharyngeal tracheal lumen airway: an assessment of airway control in the setting of upper airway hemorrhage, *Ann Emerg Med* 16:343, 1987.

Brantigan CO, Grow JB Sr: Cricothyroidotomy revisited again, *Ear Nose Throat J* 59:26-38, 1980.

Bryson TK, Benumof JL, Ward CF: The esophageal obturator airway, *Chest* 74:537, 1978.

Daily RH: Acute upper airway obstruction, *Emerg Med Clin North Am* 1:261, 1983.

Don Michael TA, Lambert EH, Mehran A: A mouth-to-lung airway for cardiac resuscitation, *Lancet* II:1329, 1968.

Don Michael TA, Lambert EH, Mehran A: The esophageal obturator airway: a new device in emergency cardiopulmonary resuscitation, *Br Med J* 281:1531, 1980.

Frass M, Frenzer R, Zdrahal F, et al: The esophageal tracheal combitube: preliminary results with a new airway for CPR, *Ann Emerg Med* 16(7):768-772, 1987.

Hardwick WC, Bluhm D: Digital intubation, *J Emerg Med* 1:317, 1984.

Iserson KV: Blind nasotracheal intubation, *Ann Emerg Med* 10(9):168-471, 1981.

Jackson C: High tracheotomy and other errors the chief causes of chronic laryngeal stenosis, *Surg Gynecol Obstet* 32:392-398, 1921.

Jordan RC: Airway management, *Emer Med Clin North Am* 6(4):671, 1988.

Kilaney SM: Complications of tracheostomy, *Ear Nose Throat J* 59:123, 1980.

Leo JD, Simon RR: Upper airway obstruction and procedures and techniques in airway management. In Brenner BE, editor: *Comprehensive management of respiratory emergencies,* Rockville, Md, 1985, Aspen Publication.

Levinson MM, Scuderi PE, Gibson RL, et al: Emergency percutaneous transtracheal ventilation (PTV), *JACEP* 8(10):396-400, 1979.

McEwen W: Clinical observations on the introduction of tracheal tubes by the mouth, instead of performing tracheotomy or laryngotomy, *Br Med J* 2:122-124, 163-165, 1880.

Meislin HW: The esophageal obturator airway: a study of respiratory effectiveness, *Ann Emerg Med* 9:54, 1980.

Niemann JT, Rosborough JP, Myers R, et al: The pharyngeotracheal lumen airway: preliminary investigation of a new adjunct, *Ann Emerg Med* 13:591-596, 1984.

Safar P, Penninck J: Cricothyroid membrane puncture with special cannula, *Anesthesiology* 28:943, 1967.

Shea SR, MacDonald JR, Gruzinski G: Prehospital endotracheal airway or esophageal gastric tube airway: a critical comparison, *Ann Emerg Med* 14:102-112, 1985.

Smith JP, Bodai BI, Auberg R, et al: A field evaluation of the esophageal obturator airway, *J Trauma* 23:317-320, 1983.

Stewart RD: Tactile orotracheal intubation, *Ann Emerg Med* 13(3):175-178, 1984.

Tintinnali JE, Claffey J: Complications of nasotracheal intubation, *Ann Emerg Med* 10(3):142-144, 1981.

Esophageal Obturator Airway (EOA)/Esophageal Gastric Tube Airway (EGTA) Insertion

EOA/EGTA insertion attempts should not exceed 30 seconds per attempt. If you are unsuccessful, hyperventilate the patient for 2 minutes and reattempt insertion.

	Possible points	Points awarded
Observe universal precautions.	1	
Hyperventilate patient with BVM.	1	
Assemble equipment, check tube and mask for cuff leaks.	2	
Lubricate tube with water-soluble jelly.	1	
Position head, pull jaw and tongue forward.	2	
Advance tube gently until mask rests on face.	1	
Ventilate patient with BVM and visualize for chest rise. Auscultate chest and epigastric area.	2	
Inflate cuff with 30 to 35 cc of air.	1	
Ventilate patient, periodically reassessing breath and epigastric sounds.	1	
TOTAL POINTS	**12**	

COMMENTS _____

_____

_____

Pharyngeal Tracheal Lumen Airway (PTL) Insertion

PTL insertion attempts should not exceed 30 seconds per attempt. If you are unsuccessful, hyperventilate the patient for 2 minutes and reattempt insertion.

Procedure	Possible points	Points awarded
Observe universal precautions.	1	
Hyperventilate patient with BVM.	1	
Test cuffs on PTL.	1	
Familiarize yourself with tube, identifying long and short tube before insertion.	1	
Lubricate tube with water-soluble jelly.	1	
Position head and pull jaw and tongue forward.	2	
Gently insert airway, advancing it to the appropriate level.	1	
Inflate both balloons simultaneously by blowing into valve.	1	
Ventilate patient through short tube and assess chest rise.	1	
Determine tracheal or esophageal position and ventilate through appropriate tube.	1	
TOTAL POINTS	**11**	

COMMENTS

Esophageal Tracheal Combitube (ETC) Insertion

ETC insertion attempts should not exceed 30 seconds per attempt. If you are unsuccessful, hyperventilate the patient for 2 minutes and reattempt insertion.

Procedure	Possible points	Points awarded
Observe universal precautions.	1	
Hyperventilate patient with BVM.	1	
Test cuffs on ETC.	1	
Familiarize yourself with tube, identifying long and short tube before insertion.	1	
Lubricate tube with water-soluble jelly.	1	
Position head and pull jaw and tongue forward.	2	
Gently insert airway, advancing it until the printed ring is aligned with teeth.	1	
Inflate line 1 (blue pilot balloon) with 100 cc of air.	1	
Inflate line 2 (white pilot balloon) with approximately 15 ml of air.	1	
Ventilate the patient through the longer blue tube and assess chest rise and breath/espigastric sounds.	1	
Determine tracheal or esophageal position and ventilate through appropriate tube.	1	
TOTAL POINTS	**12**	

COMMENTS _____

_____

_____

Endotracheal Intubation (Adult)

Intubation attempts should not exceed 30 seconds per attempt. If unsuccessful after two attempts, the paramedic should consider alternate airway management techniques. The patient must be hyperventilated between intubation attempts.

Procedure	Possible points	Points awarded
Observe universal precautions.	1	
Hyperventilate patient with BVM.	1	
Assemble laryngoscope blade and handle.	1	
Check light operation.	1	
Prepare ETT tape, and assemble other needed equipment.	2	
Insert stylet into ETT.	1	
Position head in sniffing position.	1	
Insert laryngoscope in right side of mouth and move tongue to left.	1	
Visualize (and verbalize) epiglottis and vocal cords.	1	
Properly insert ETT.	1	
Remove laryngoscope, stabilize tube, and remove stylet.	3	
Inflate cuff with 5 to 10cc of air.	1	
Ventilate patient with BVM; assess breath and epigastric sounds.	1	
Secure tube.	1	
Reconfirm tube placement after securing.	1	
TOTAL POINTS	**18**	

COMMENTS _____

_____

_____

Nasotracheal Intubation

Nasotracheal intubation is a procedure used when intubating patients with spontaneous respiration. This procedure should be completed within 2 minutes; however, it requires gentle technique to successfully accomplish.

Procedure	Possible points	Points awarded
Observe universal precautions.	1	
Select appropriate size ETT and test cuff.	1	
Lubricate tube with lidocaine jelly. Form "circle" with tube to shape it.	2	
Anesthetize nostrils and pharynx with spray anesthesia (if time allows).	1	
Gently insert tube into the nares and into nasopharynx. Continue to slide the tube down until vapor appears in the tube or breath sounds are heard.	2	
Listen closely for breath sounds. Insert tube into trachea during patient inspiration, advancing tube until the adapter meets nares.	2	
Confirm placement of tube.	1	
Secure tube as necessary.	1	
TOTAL POINTS	**11**	

COMMENTS _____

_____

_____

Surgical Cricothyrotomy

Surgical cricothyrotomy is only indicated when the paramedic is unable to secure an airway by other non-invasive procedures.

Procedure	Possible points	Points awarded
Observe universal precautions.	1	
Hyperventilate patient if possible.	1	
Open cricothyrotomy kit and prepare equipment (select ETT).	1	
Surgically prep neck with povidone-iodine swabs.	1	
Drape area with fenestrated sheet.	1	
Orient yourself to landmarks of neck, and stabilize thyroid cartilage.	2	
Make traverse incision over cricothyroid membrane, sponging bleeding as necessary.	1	
Feel cricothyroid membrane. Carefully make horizontal incision over lower part of the membrane.	1	
Insert scalpel handle into incision and rotate it 90 degrees, opening the airway.	2	
Insert ETT or tracheostomy tube into opening	1	
Inflate cuff and ventilate patient.	2	
Observe chest rise and fall; auscultate breath and epigastric sounds.	2	
Secure tube in place.	1	
TOTAL POINTS	**17**	

COMMENTS _____

_____

_____

Precutaneous Transtracheal Ventilation (Needle Cricothyrotomy)

In situations where endotracheal intubation is not possible, the needle cricothyrotomy is a valuable alternative, and is safer than the surgical cricothyrotomy.

Procedure	Possible points	Points awarded
Observe universal precautions.	1	
Hyperventilate patient if possible.	1	
Orient yourself to landmarks of neck, locating cricothyroid membrane.	1	
Surgically prep area with povidone-iodine swabs.	1	
Remove hub from 12- or 14-gauge over-the-needle catheter. Attach 10-cc syringe to catheter. Also, prepare Y-connector apparatus.	2	
Relocate cricothyroid membrane and puncture skin with needle.	1	
Advance needle at 45-degree angle caudally and push needle until it "pops" into the trachea.	2	
Advance catheter from needle into the trachea, removing needle.	1	
Confirm placement of catheter.	1	
Secure catheter.	1	
Attach three-way stopcock to hub of catheter.	1	
Connect Y-connector apparatus to catheter and oxygen source.	2	
Ventilate patient, using 1:4 ratio.	1	
TOTAL POINTS	**16**	

COMMENTS _____

_____

_____

Tracheal Suctioning of the Nonintubated Patient

Tracheal suctioning in the absence of an ETT can result in anatomical damage, bleeding, and additional airway obstruction if this procedure is not performed delicately.

Procedure	Possible points	Points awarded
Observe universal precautions.	1	
Position patient.	1	
Preoxygenate patient.	1	
Open catheter kit and prepare equipment, including sterile gloves.	1	
Gently insert catheter through nostril into pharynx, without engaging suction.	1	
Ask patient to assume the sniffing position, if possible.	1	
Advance catheter into larynx during inspiration. Proceed through vocal cords during coughing or inspiration.	1	
Once in trachea, engage suction intermittently and withdraw catheter using a rotating motion.	1	
Reoxygenate patient.	1	
TOTAL POINTS	9	

COMMENTS _____

_____

_____

Tracheal Suctioning of the Intubated Patient

Tracheal suctioning can accomplished via an ETT if the patient is intubated. Suctioning an ET tube should last no longer than 5 seconds.

Procedure	Possible points	Points awarded
Observe universal precautions.	1	
Preoxygenate patient.	1	
Confirm EKG monitoring.	1	
Open catheter kit and prepare equipment, including sterile gloves.	1	
Introduce catheter into ETT without touching outside of the tube.	1	
Advance catheter as far as possible, without engaging suction.	1	
Engage intermittent suction and withdraw catheter, using a rotating motion.	1	
Reoxygenate patient.	1	
TOTAL POINTS	**8**	

COMMENTS _____

_____

_____

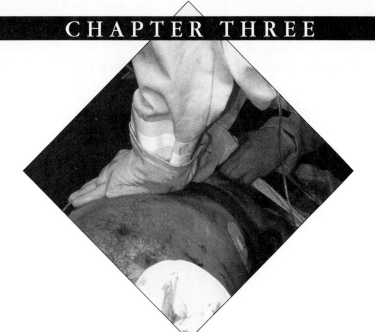

CHAPTER THREE

Circulatory Management

Objectives

A paramedic should be able to—

1. Define tension pneumothorax.

2. List four common causes of tension pneumothorax.

3. List eight clinical signs of tension pneumothorax.

4. State the technique used for decompression of tension pneumothorax.

5. Demonstrate thoracic decompression using a decompression mannequin or acceptable simulator.

6. Discuss two mechanisms of action of the pneumatic antishock garment.

7. List five indications for application of the pneumatic antishock garment.

8. List two absolute contraindications for application of the pneumatic antishock garment.

9. List five relative contraindications for application of the pneumatic antishock garment.

10. List three techniques of application of the pneumatic antishock garment.

11. State the main reason for deflating the pneumatic antishock garment in the field.

12. Demonstrate the three procedures for application of the pneumatic antishock garment.

13. Demonstrate the technique for deflation of the pneumatic antishock garment.

14. Define peripheral intravenous cannulation.

15. List the two common indications for peripheral intravenous cannulation in the field.

16. Name the most common location of intravenous cannula.

17. List the equipment items necessary for peripheral intravenous cannulation.

18. List the steps involved in the initiation of intravenous cannulation.

19. Demonstrate the proper technique of peripheral intravenous cannulation using a cannulation model.

20. State the anatomic location of the external jugular vein.

21. List the indication for using the external jugular vein for intravenous cannulation.

22. List the steps involved in the initiation of external jugular vein cannulation.

23. Identify the external jugular vein on a live model.

24. Demonstrate the proper technique of external jugular vein cannulation in a cadaver laboratory or emergency department under the supervision of a physician.

Photo courtesy Colin Williams/*Emergency.*

Case Scenario

On arrival at the scene of a domestic quarrel, police advise you that a 28-year-old male who has been shot with a .38 Special is lying on the floor of his residence. They have the wife (and weapon) in custody.

Copious bleeding has occurred from a wound to the patient's chest, just under the right nipple. While approaching, snoring sounds are heard and you see blood "blow" from the hole in the patient's chest with each breath. He does not respond to your voice. You immediately seal the opening on three sides using a defibrillator pad and 3-inch tape, and you have your partner begin hyperventilation with a bag-valve-mask with high flow oxygen. Breath sounds are decreased bilaterally, yet "noisy" on the right. Carotid pulse is rapid and weak, radial is absent; capillary refill is 4-seconds; he fails to respond to verbal or painful stimuli.

The pneumatic antishock garment is applied with only the legs inflated. The patient is secured to a long spineboard.

En route to the trauma center, the patient is intubated with a No. 8 endotracheal tube, and two large-bore intravenous lines (IVs) of lactated Ringer's are initiated. After a detailed assessment, you note that the breath sounds on the left are now absent, the trachea is deviated to the right, the jugular veins are distended, and the patient is very difficult to ventilate. The decision is made to perform a thoracic needle decompression to evac-

uate the air that has built up in the left chest cavity. Successful placement of a 14-gauge catheter results in immediate alleviation of the patient's symptomatology. He is delivered to the emergency department with marked improvement, where a chest tube is placed by the receiving physician.

The skills discussed in this chapter on circulatory management range from the basic (pneumatic antishock garment application), to the advanced (chest decompression). As with all EMS skills, the success of the paramedics who use these procedures depends on practice and retention. Not all systems will use all of these skills.

It should also be noted that several skills addressed are not isolated to just circulatory system management. For example, thoracic decompression is a management skill of both the respiratory and circulatory system.

◆ Pneumatic Antishock Garment Application

The pneumatic antishock garment (PASG) surrounds the lower extremities and abdomen and is used to control bleeding, increase perfusion to vital organs, and splint the pelvis and/or lower extremities.

Background

The PASG has many names, but most commonly is called the pneumatic antishock garment, or medical or military antishock trousers (MAST). It is most commonly used to treat hypotension following trauma. The device increases peripheral vascular resistance, but only autotransfuses cephalad approximately 250 ml of blood from the lower extremities and the abdomen in the adult.

Indications

- Hypovolemic shock
- Other causes of shock for which MAST may be helpful: spinal shock, overdose, septic shock, anaphylaxis
- Intraabdominal or gastrointestinal bleeding, ruptured aortic abdominal aneurysm
- Stabilization of pelvic or lower extremity fractures
- Compression of external bleeding

Contraindications

- Absolute
  - Pulmonary edema
  - Congestive heart failure
- Relative
  - Abdominal injuries with protruding abdominal contents
  - Cardiogenic shock
  - Impaled objects to the leg or abdomen
  - Lumbar spine instability—use lower extremity compartments only
  - Penetrating thoracic injuries
  - Pregnancy—use lower extremity compartments only during third trimester
  - Isolated head trauma
  - Use legs only with pediatric patients

When a patient's respiratory condition becomes markedly worse after inflation, consider diaphragmatic rupture or tension pneumothorax. Deflation under medical direction/control should be considered.

The Pros and Cons of the Pneumatic Antishock Garment

The use of MAST in prehospital care has recently generated much controversy. A 1988 article by McSwain reviewed 215 papers published in medical journals. The author concluded that multiple studies have demonstrated that the PASG does "improve blood pressure, control hemorrhage, improve carotid and upper body blood flow, improve the ability of prehospital providers to start IV lines, and improve survival (particularly short term) with few hospital and even fewer prehospital complications. The device produces its blood pressure response by improving preload, increasing systemic vascular resistance, and mobilizing some blood (500 to 1000 ml) to the upper body compartment above the device." However, studies indicate that quantities as little as 150 to 300 ml are autotransfused.

The use of MAST for hypovolemic shock from penetrating trauma has been challenged in studies from Mattox and colleagues in Houston. Major conclusions from these studies were:

1. "... for penetrating trauma with prehospital times of 30 minutes or less, MAST provides no advantage with regard to survival, length of stay, or reduced hospital costs." (Mattox, Bickell, Pepe, et al: *J Trauma*, 1986.)
2. "... the PASG provides no significant advantage in improving survival in the urban prehospital management of penetrating abdominal injuries." (Bickell, Pepe, Bailey et al: *Ann Emerg Med*, 1987.)
3. "MAST application adversely affected the outcome most significantly for patients with cardiac and thoracic vascular injury." (Mattox, Bickell, Pepe, et al, *J Trauma*, 1989)

These studies came from a single urban EMS system with paramedic ambulances, short transport times, and one easily accessible trauma center. The conclusions should be considered in that context. No similar studies have been performed for rural EMS systems, nor have blunt injuries been taken into consideration.

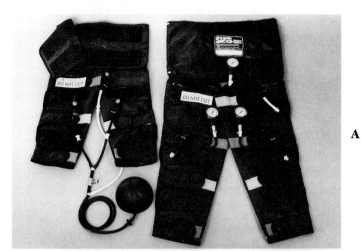

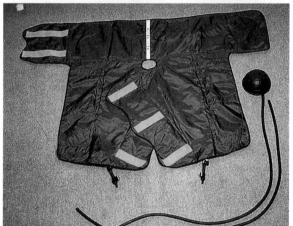

Figure 3-1 **A**, Jobst pediatric trousers (without gauges) and adult trousers (with gauges). (Courtesy The Jobst Institute, Inc.) **B**, David Clark trousers (without gauges). (Courtesy David Clark Co.)

PEARLS & PITFALLS

Gauges, Gauges, and More Gauges

Monitoring the patient's vital signs is more important than monitoring pressure gauges on models of PASG that have them. Changes in level of consciousness, heart rate, and blood pressure provide you with more useful information than what the pressure is inside of the pneumatic antishock garment. Remember: the patient is in shock, not the garment!

Equipment

Two major types of PASG devices are available. One type has pressure gauges for monitoring the suit pressure (Figure 3-1, *A*), whereas the other type has pop-off valves that limit pressures to approximately 106 mm Hg (Figure 3-1, *B*).

Procedure: methods of application and inflation

1. There are three methods to apply the PASG. The *logroll* method is most commonly used when a spinal injury is suspected and at least three team members are available to properly logroll the patient. The garment should be fan-folded, or layered, and placed next to the patient (Figure 3-2). The cervical area and head are protected by one member, while a

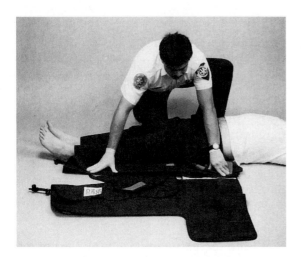

Figure 3-2 Patient is logrolled onto his side, and the fanfolded garment is pulled into place.

minimum of two others support the body and roll the patient onto the rescuer's knees. The garment is then slid into place, under the patient and just inferior to the twelfth rib. The patient is then rolled as a unit onto the garment, and the velcro is secured. Careful alignment of the velcro straps will prevent the straps from popping loose during inflation.

The second method is the *diaper* method, which consists of simply placing the garment flat, in the open position, at the feet of the supine patient (Figure 3-3, *A*). Two team members simultaneously lift the legs, slide the garment up under the patient, and lower the legs onto the garment. The hips are then lifted, and the garment slid up just inferior to the twelfth rib (Figure 3-3, *B*). The garment is wrapped around the patient, and the velcro secured.

The third method is the *trouser* method and can be performed two ways. To begin, open the trousers and attach the velcro in the wide-open position, creating a very large pair of pants (Figure 3-4). One team member can place an arm up each leg of the garment, or more easily, two rescuers can place one arm each (one right arm, one left arm) up the respective leg of the garment. Next, place a hand over the patient's foot, lift the legs, and slide the garment off onto the patient's extremities.

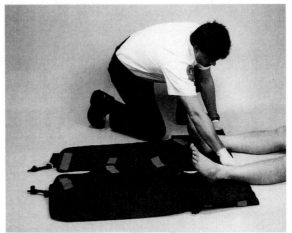

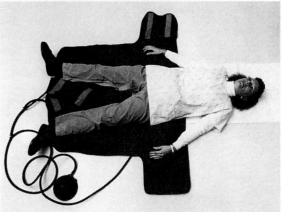

Figure 3-3 **A**, When using the diaper method, the PASG is unfolded flat and pulled under the patient. **B**, Position the patient supine, with the garment just below the twelfth rib.

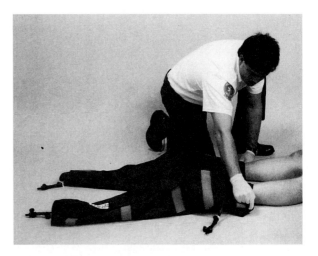

Figure 3-4 The trouser method can be prefolded and stored in the box, simply by barely touching the velcro strips.

Lower the legs and move up to the pelvis. Lift the pelvis slightly and slide the abdominal section up under the torso, just inferior to the twelfth rib and secure as previously described (Figure 3-5, *A* to *C*).

2. Once the garment is secured, attach the tubing-foot pump apparatus to the trousers.

3. Open all stopcock valves so that all three compartments can be inflated simultaneously. (Some areas will require that the leg compartments be inflated first, then the abdominal section.)

4. Inflate the garment, using the foot pump, until the velcro crackles, air exhausts through the "pop-off" valves, and/or the patient's blood pressure exceeds a systolic pressure of 100 mm Hg (Figure 3-6).

5. Close all stopcocks. (The foot pump should remain attached and stay with the patient until the garment is removed.)

6. Monitor the patient for hemodynamic and respiratory changes, as well as air leakage from the garment.

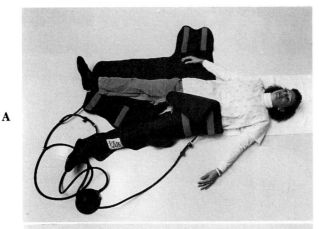

A

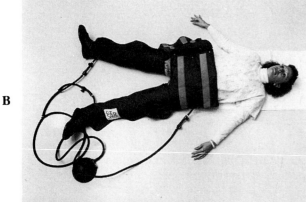

B

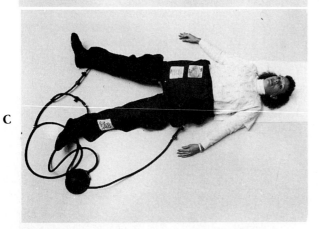

C

Figure 3-5 A, The left leg of the garment is wrapped around the patient's left leg. Velcro is secured. **B,** Right leg of the garment is wrapped around the patient's right leg. Velcro is secured. **C,** The abdominal compartment is then wrapped around the abdomen and secured.

PEARLS
&
PITFALLS

Just a Reminder...

Practicing the application of the PASG with your partner will markedly decrease application time. If the patient is in shock from trauma, quickly examine the abdomen, pelvis and legs for injury just prior to application. The PASG is particularly beneficial for stabilizing pelvic and lower extremity fractures. Bone alignment occurs and bleeding is often tamponaded by the direct pressure of the garment. A well-practiced team should be able to examine the lower half of the body and apply the PASG in less than 2 minutes.

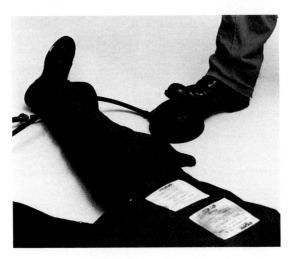

Figure 3-6 Inflate the trousers using the foot pump until after the velcro has seated itself or the patient's systolic pressure is adequate.

Procedure: deflation and removal

1. Evaluate the patient's vital signs and verify the patient's stability.

2. Ensure that IV lines are accessible, that the patient has received proper volume, and that support teams such as a surgical crew are available.

3. Check the garment to ensure that the foot pump is still attached (in case the need arises to rapidly reinflate) and that all stopcocks are in the closed position.

4. Remove the abdominal hose and open the stopcock for approximately 2 seconds, releasing about one third of the pressure in the abdominal section. Close the stopcock.

5. Reevaluate vital signs and, if no significant change occurs, continue the procedure until deflated. A rule-of-thumb is that a rise in heart rate of 5 beats per minute or a drop in blood pressure of 5 mm Hg represents a significant change. If an increase in heart rate or drop in systolic pressure occurs, cease the deflation procedure and open the IV lines. An infusion of 250 ml of lactated Ringer's or normal saline serves as a fluid challenge.

6. Repeat steps 4 and 5 with each leg until the garment is fully deflated. It may take up to 30 minutes to properly remove the PASG.

Miscellaneous Tips

• The PASG may be placed "prophylactically" on a patient when the mechanism indicates potential injury, even though the vital signs do not demonstrate shock. If signs of shock appear, you are then prepared to inflate the trousers.
• Inflation of the PASG will frequently make peripheral veins distend, thus making IV insertion easier.
• If a patient is to be flown by helicopter or non-pressured aircraft, altitude may increase PASG pressures. Monitor the garment and lower extremities of your patient.

Respiratory Distress Following PASG Application

Deflation of the PASG is generally reserved for the controlled environment of the emergency department. Occasionally though, deflation in the field must be considered when a patient develops respiratory distress following inflation of the garment. If time permits, you should consult Medical Control/Direction for advice. However, if the distress is severe and the patient is decompensating, take immediate action. Deflate the abdominal section of the garment and monitor the patient closely. This deflation procedure is usually guided by local or state protocol.

◆ Peripheral Intravenous Cannulation

Intravenous cannulation is the process of placing a catheter (metal or plastic) into a peripheral vein for the administration of fluids or drugs.

Background

Peripheral intravenous cannulation provides access to the circulation for rapid administration of fluids and drugs. Commonly, peripheral intravenous cannulation is used for fluid administration in shock and as a lifeline for various medical conditions such as cardiac disease, hypoglycemia, and seizures. Intravenous cannulation in the field is most commonly performed with a plastic catheter inserted over a hollow needle. Other types of cannulas are hollow needles and plastic catheters inserted through a hollow needle.

Indication

Intravenous cannulation is indicated for the administration of drugs or fluids in any critically ill or potentially critically ill patient.

Contraindications

Although there are no true absolute contraindications, peripheral intravenous cannulation should not significantly delay scene times.

Intravenous cannulation in most patients should be started while en route to the hospital when possible.

Equipment (Figure 3-7)

- Intravenous fluid ordered (e.g., lactated Ringer's, normal saline, or dextrose 5% in water)
- Intravenous infusion set—use microdrip tubing for lifelines used for drug administration, and macrodrip tubing for rapid fluid administration
- Intravenous catheter (cannula)—preferably 18 gauge for lifelines and 12 to 16 gauge for fluid administration
- Povidone-iodine or alcohol preps
- Sterile dressing (e.g., 4×4 gauze pad)
- Adhesive tape strips, 3 to 4 inches in length
- 10 cc syringe, vacutainer tubes for blood samples
- Tourniquet (commercial or blood pressure cuff)
- Armboard
- Latex gloves

Procedure

1. Explain to the patient the need for intravenous cannulation and describe what you'll be doing.

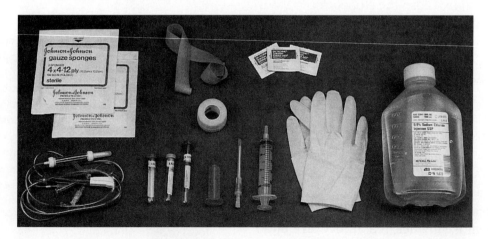

Figure 3-7 Peripheral intravenous cannulation equipment.

2. Observe universal precautions (glove minimally).

3. Place a commercial tourniquet or inflate a blood pressure cuff just above the elbow and place the arm in a dependent position (Figure 3-8). If using a blood pressure cuff, inflate until 20 mm Hg below the systolic pressure.

4. Select a prominent vein by feel more than sight. Choose the most distal prominent vein on the hand, forearm, or antecubital space that is straight, on a flat surface, and not rolling. If possible, avoid veins over joints, using the antecubital veins as a last resort.

5. A vein may be distended for easier cannulation by gently tapping on it with your fingers.

6. Prep the venipuncture site with povidone-iodine or alcohol prep, using a firm circular motion from the vein outward (Figure 3-9).

7. With traction on the skin below the venipuncture site, stabilize the vein.

8. Tell the patient there will be a quick, painful stick.

9. With the bevel of the needle upward, puncture the skin using a 30- to 45-degree angle. Enter the vein directly from above or from the side (Figure 3-10).

10. When the vein is entered, you should feel a "pop" and see blood return through the catheter.

11. Carefully lower the catheter and advance the needle and catheter approximately 2 mm to stabilize the needle in the vein.

12. Slide the catheter off of the needle into the vein and then remove the needle (Figure 3-11). Dispose of the needle into a puncture-proof (sharps) container. Do not attempt to recap the needle.

13. Consider drawing a blood sample using a syringe or luer-adapter and vacutainer.

14. Release the tourniquet (Figure 3-12) and attach the infusion tubing to the hub of the catheter (Figure 3-13).

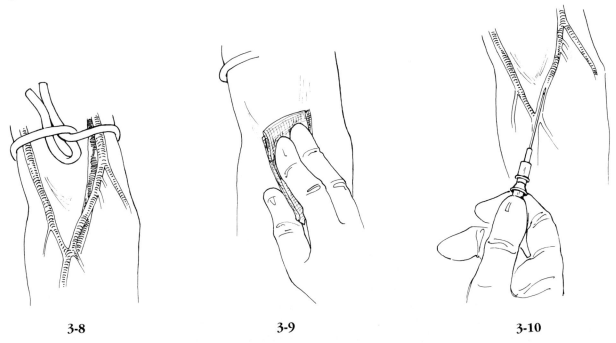

3-8   3-9   3-10

Figure 3-8   Venous tourniquet placed just proximal to the antecubital area.
Figure 3-9   Cleanse the skin with alcohol or povidone-iodine, using a circular motion.
Figure 3-10   With the bevel of the needle upward, puncture the skin and enter the vein either from on top or from the side of the vein.

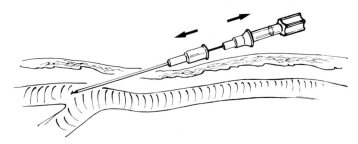

Figure 3-11 Slide the catheter over the needle into the vein and then remove the needle.

15. Open the flow regulator on the IV tubing. The fluid should run freely.

16. Cover the venipuncture site with povidone-iodine ointment.

17. Tape the catheter to the skin, using any acceptable technique.

18. Make a loop with the infusion tubing and tape the loop to the arm. This will allow a little extra tubing in case the IV bag is accidentally pulled away from the patient.

19. If the vein is near or over a joint, immobilize it with an armboard to prevent dislodgement of the catheter.

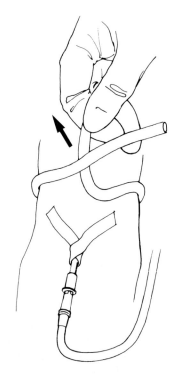

Figure 3-12 Release the tourniquet.

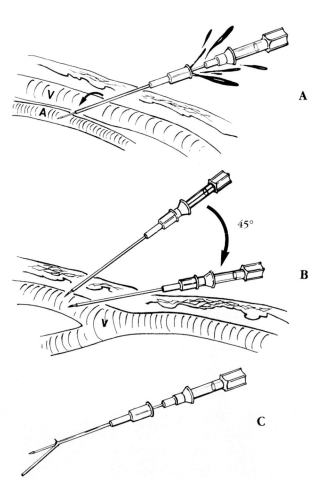

Figure 3-14 **A,** Inadvertent arterial cannulation with bright red blood spurting through the catheter. **B,** A sharp angle of insertion will cause the needle to go into the vein and through the other side. **C,** Over-the-needle catheter shear can occur when the needle is partially withdrawn and then reinserted.

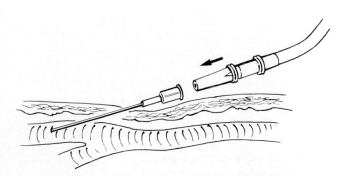

Figure 3-13 Attach the infusion tubing to the catheter.

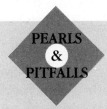

PEARLS
&
PITFALLS

Complications of Intravenous Therapy

There are many complications that can develop with intravenous therapy. Some complications can be easily corrected in the field, while others may require the discontinuance of the IV catheter. Discussed below are some of the more common problems seen by prehospital care providers.

- *Misidentification of a vessel:* Be careful that the vessel you have chosen does not have a pulsation, indicating it is probably an artery. If arterial cannulation does occur bright red blood will spurt intermittently through the catheter (Figure 3-14, *A*). In this case, remove the catheter and apply direct pressure for 5 minutes with a gloved hand and dressing.

- *Infiltration:* Intravenous solution infiltrating into subcutaneous tissue is common when catheters become dislodged. Edema, pain, decrease in the infusion rate and failure to get blood return in the tubing when the IV solution is held below the level of the heart are all signs of infiltration. Stop the infusion and remove the catheter. Some medications, such as D_{50} can cause tissue necrosis.

- *Incorrect angle of insertion:* A sharp angle (greater than 45 degrees) of insertion will cause the needle to go into the vein and through the other side, resulting in infiltration (Figure 3-14, *B*).

- *Catheter shear:* Over the needle catheters can shear. Needles that are partially withdrawn and then reinserted can result in catheter shear. The sheared part of the catheter becomes a potential embolus when it breaks loose into the blood stream. **Never** reinsert a partially withdrawn needle (Figure 3-14, *C*).

- *Run-away IVs:* After you have opened the clamp to check that the fluid is running without difficulty, make sure you adjust the infusion rate. Many patients receive accidental fluid overloads secondary to run-away IVs. This can be life threatening in a patient with acute pulmonary edema.

- *Poor catheter position:* Some IVs that cease flowing can be corrected by making a small change in the position of the catheter. This may require that you remove some of the tape, readjust the position, and then resecuring the catheter.

- *Hard-to-locate veins:* Many patients will present with poor vascular status. Locating a vein in these patients may present a major problem, especially if you are in a life-threatening situation. Blood pressure cuffs are frequently more successful as tourniquets than commercial types. On the other hand, if your patient is obese, place one tourniquet at the wrist and another just above the elbow. This will allow blood to pool between the two tourniquets and help the vein to pop up. IV drug abusers and patients with vascular disease, such as diabetes, often have extremely difficult veins to cannulate. Ask the patient where to look for your best stick. Consider the external jugular as a alternate site.

- *Rapid volume replacement:* Pressure bags on intravenous solutions and elevation of the IV bags increase the rate of fluid administration, as indicated for the treatment of shock. In addition, the use of a short (1 ¼-inch catheter) will accelerate fluid flow.

- *Injection:* One of the most common complications seen as the result of prehospital IVs is infection. Although field conditions are not always the most sanitary, every effort should be made to use aseptic technique. A combination of povidone-iodine and alcohol is recommended.

♦ External Jugular Vein Cannulation

The external jugular vein is a large vessel in the neck that may be used by paramedics for intravenous cannulation. This vein is considered to be a peripheral IV site.

Background

The external jugular vein runs from behind the angle of the jaw downward across the sternocleidomastoid muscle to pierce the fascia above the middle third of the clavicle. It joins the subclavian vein just behind the clavicle (Figure 3-15, *A* and *B*). If EMS systems allow the procedure, external jugular vein cannulation can be used anytime peripheral intravenous cannulation is required.

Indication

External jugular vein cannulation is indicated in a patient who requires peripheral intravenous cannulation in whom an extremity vein cannot be catheterized.

Contraindications

- Obscured landmarks caused by local trauma, hematoma, or subcutaneous emphysema
- Cervical collar

Equipment

- Fluid ordered (e.g., lactated Ringer's, normal saline, or dextrose 5% in water)
- Intravenous infusion set—use microdrip tubing for lifelines and for drug administration and macrodrip tubing for rapid fluid administration

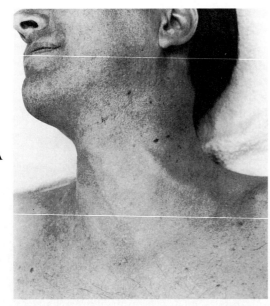

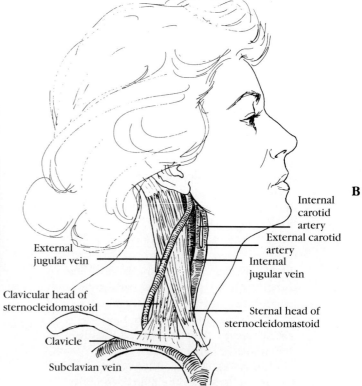

Figure 3-15 **A,** The external jugular vein crosses the sternocleidomastoid muscle. **B,** The external jugular vein runs from behind the angle of the jaw, downward across the sternocleidomastoid muscle, to pierce the fascia above the middle third of the clavicle. The internal carotid artery and internal jugular vein are medial to the muscle.

- IV extension tubing
- IV catheter (cannula)—preferably 18 gauge for lifelines and 12 to 16 gauge for fluid administration
- Povidone-iodine prep
- Sterile dressing (e.g., 4×4 gauze pad)
- Adhesive tape strips, 3 to 4 inches length
- 10-cc syringe, vacutainers for blood samples
- Sterile gloves

Procedure

1. Explain procedure to patient.
2. Use universal precautions.
3. Position the patient supine with feet elevated.
4. Turn the head in the direction away from the side to be cannulated.
5. Prep the skin with povidone-iodine.
6. Apply traction on the vein just above the clavicle.
7. Attach a 10-cc syringe to an IV catheter. Align the catheter and point the tip of the catheter toward the feet.
8. Tell the patient there will be a quick, painful stick.

9. With the bevel of the needle upward, puncture the skin using a 30-degree angle. The needle tip should enter midway between the angle of the jaw and the clavicle, and should be aimed toward the shoulder on the same side as the vein. Apply suction to the syringe. As you enter the vein, you'll note a flashback of blood (Figure 3-16).
10. Carefully lower the catheter and advance the needle and catheter approximately 2 mm to stabilize the needle in the vein.
11. Slide the catheter off of the needle into the vein and then remove the needle. Dispose of needle and syringe into a puncture proof container. Don't attempt to recap the needle.
12. Consider drawing a blood sample using a syringe or luer-adapter and vacutainer.
13. Attach the infusion tubing to the hub of the catheter.
14. Open the flow regulator on the IV tubing. The fluid should run freely.
15. Cover the site with povidone-iodine ointment.
16. Tape the catheter to the skin using any acceptable technique (Figure 3-17).
17. Make a loop with the infusion tubing and tape the loop to the neck so there will be extra tubing in case the IV bag is accidentally pulled away from the patient. Never use cir-

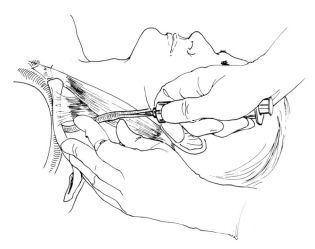

Figure 3-16 Turn the head away from the side that you wish to cannulate. Pull tension with one finger on the vein just above the clavicle. Align the catheter and pierce the skin, entering midway between the angle of the jaw and the clavicle.

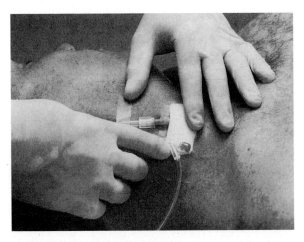

Figure 3-17 Tape the catheter to the skin using any acceptable method.

External Jugular Cannulation

Paramedics often hesitate to use the external jugular vein because it is in the neck, close to the carotid artery and other vital structures. Although it is prudent to be cautious, remember that the external jugular vein is frequently larger, more easily identified, and may be easier to cannulate than other vessels.

Pressure and tension on the external jugular vein just above the clavicle will distend the vein markedly and make cannulation easier.

cumferential taping because of vascular compromise that can result in a decreased cerebral circulation.

◆ Thoracic Decompression

Thoracic decompression is placement of a needle through the chest wall of a patient whose lung has collapsed as a result of a one-way valve air leak.

Background

Recognition of tension pneumothorax is facilitated by understanding that it results from a one-way valve air leak from the lung and/or through the chest wall. Air enters one side of the thoracic cavity without any means of escape, thus producing total collapse of the lung on the affected side and pressure against the mediastinum and lung on the uninvolved side (Figure 3-18, *A* to *C*). The rise in intrapleural pressure decreases venous return to the heart and decreases cardiac output. Ventilation and perfusion are rapidly compromised. This is a life-threatening condition that will result in

death if not recognized and treated rapidly. It occurs most commonly in the clinical settings of chest trauma and in manually or mechanically ventilated patients with chronic lung disease.

The initial signs of tension pneumothorax may be subtle, such as restlessness. However, these patients have an extremely rapid downhill course over a period of just a few minutes. The clinical signs of tension pneumothorax are listed below.

Common Causes of Tension Pneumothorax

- Mechanical ventilation
- Spontaneous pneumothorax from ruptured emphysematous blebs
- Chest trauma, blunt or penetrating
- Fractured rib(s) or flail sternum secondary to chest compressions

Clinical Signs of Tension Pneumothorax

- Restlessness and agitation
- Increased airway resistance on ventilating patient
- Neck vein distention
- Respiratory distress—severe dyspnea, tachypnea, air hunger in the conscious patient
- Unilateral absence of breath sounds on affected side
- Hyperresonance to percussion on affected side
- Hypotension
- Cyanosis
- Tracheal deviation toward unaffected side
- Respiratory arrest

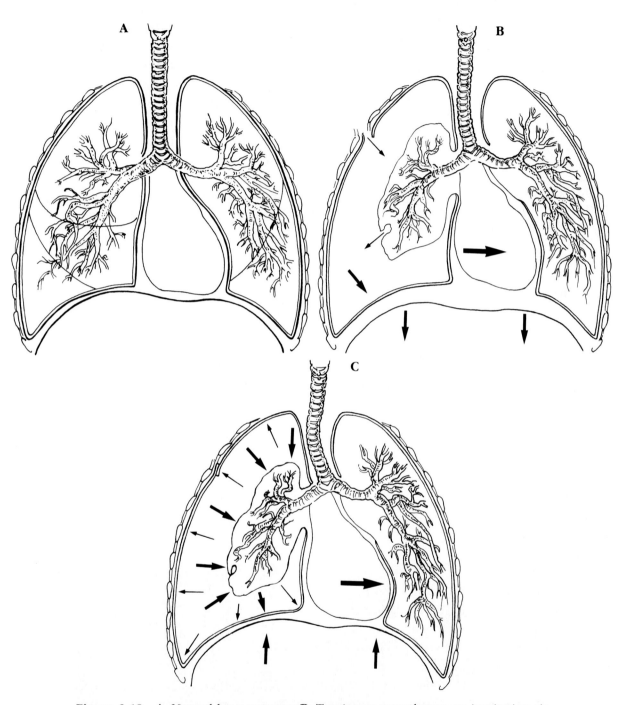

Figure 3-18 **A**, Normal lung anatomy. **B**, Tension pneumothorax: on inspiration air leaks into the pleural cavity from the punctured lung or chest wall. **C**, Tension pneumothorax: on expiration there is no escape for the increasing volume of air on the affected side.

The Need for Speed...

From the time of onset of a tension pneumothorax until needle decompression is performed, speed is of paramount importance. If clinical signs of tension pneumothorax are present, proceed with needle decompression immediately or as soon as your protocols permit. Commonly, the first sign of tension pneumothorax in intubated patients is a decreased ability to ventilate, recognized when it becomes much harder to squeeze the bag. Although tracheal deviation is listed as a sign of tension pneumothorax in all major textbooks, this sign is actually a late finding and not commonly seen in the field.

A high index of suspicion and repeated assessment in patients with clinical profiles at risk for tension pneumothorax are extremely important. Although tension pneumothorax is not an everyday experience for a paramedic, its prompt recognition and treatment are dramatically lifesaving.

Indication

Thoracic decompression is indicated in patients with clinical signs and symptoms consistent with tension pneumothorax.

Contraindications

There are no contraindications for performing a needle decompression for patients meeting the above criteria; however, medical direction/control may be required in your locale before executing this skill.

Equipment (Figure 3-19)

- Large-bore over-the-needle catheter (14-gauge or larger)
- 10-cc syringe
- Povidone-iodine preps
- Finger cut from a sterile glove for flutter valve (alternatively, a Heimlich flutter valve may be used)
- Sterile dressing
- Sterile gloves
- (McSwain Dart is used in some systems)

Procedure

1. Observe universal precautions (gloves and eye protection).

2. Cleanse the chest on the side of decreased breath sounds using povidone-iodine solution.

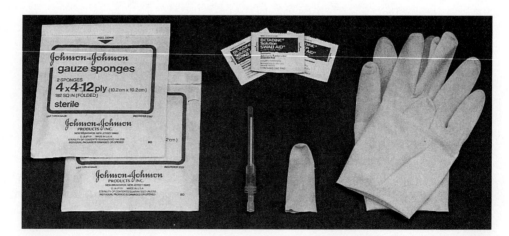

Figure 3-19 Equipment needed to decompress a pneumothorax: large-bore, over-the-needle catheter; povidone-iodine; finger cut from sterile glove; sterile dressing

Things Aren't Always As Easy As They Look

Although training in hospital and laboratory settings gives the paramedic an idea of how to perform a procedure, there still is nothing like the field for seeing how it really works... or doesn't work! Remember that things do not always go in the field as practiced in the classroom. Listed below are three possible complications to consider.

The paramedic should be aware that ambient noise on the scene or during transport may compromise the ability to hear the "hiss" commonly heard on successful needle decompression. Thus, you may have to depend on how it feels when the needle "pops" into the thoracic cavity and then evaluate your patient.

If breath sounds are unequal in the intubated patient, make sure you check for possible endotracheal tube placement in the mainstem bronchus before assuming the patient has a tension pneumothorax.

Don't waste much time preparing the surgical glove finger-catheter apparatus. If you're having trouble, eliminate the surgical glove finger and just use the catheter alone. You may be able to control the air flow by using your gloved thumb.

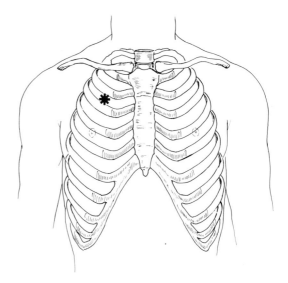

Figure 3-20 Landmark for decompression just above third rib in midclavicular line on affected side.

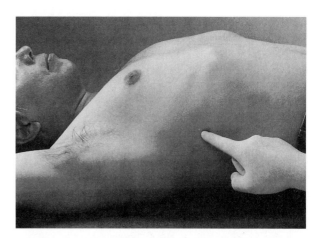

Figure 3-21 Landmark for decompression just above sixth rib in midaxillary line on affected side.

3. Attach a 10-cc syringe to a 14-gauge (or larger) over-the-needle catheter. Puncture the skin perpendicularly just superior to the third rib (second intercostal space) in the midclavicular line (approximately in line with the nipple) until the thoracic cavity is entered (Figure 3-20, Figure 3-22, *A*). In the presence of a suspected hemothorax, the fifth intercostal space in the midaxillary line can be used to evacuate air and allow for drainage of pleural blood (Figure 3-21).

4. On entering the thoracic cavity with a tension pneumothorax, you should feel a pop, and then, depending on the level of ambient noise, you may hear a "hiss" as air is decompressed (Figure 3-22, *B*). Alternately, you may see the plunger of the syringe push outward.

5. Advance the catheter and remove the needle (Figure 3-22, *C*).

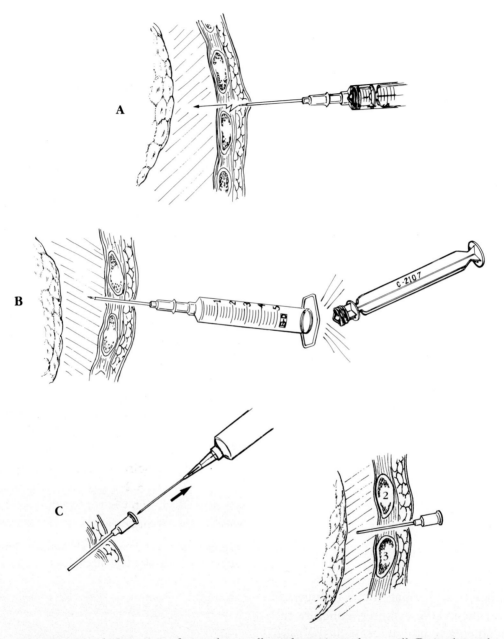

Figure 3-22 **A**, Insertion of over-the-needle catheter into chest wall. **B**, As the catheter enters the pleural cavity, the tension produced by large amounts of air in the thoracic cavity is suddenly released. If the catheter is attached to a syringe, the pressure may "pop" the plunger out of the syringe. **C**, Advance the catheter until the hub touches the chest wall; then remove the needle.

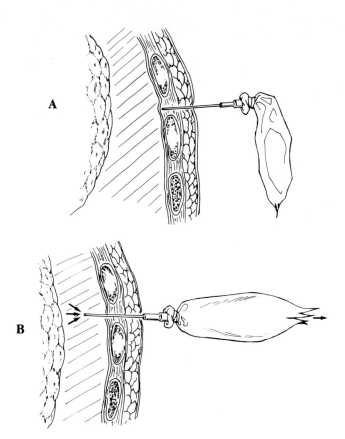

Figure 3-23 **A**, Flutter valve collapsed during inspiration; **B**, flutter valve open during expiration.

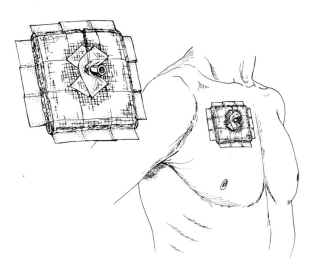

Figure 3-24 Catheter is secured to the chest wall with dressing and tape.

The Successful Decompression

On successful needle decompression there should be an immediate, marked improvement in the patient's condition. However, the paramedic must be aware that, even with successful decompression, clinical signs may recur on the same side within minutes. If this occurs, simply perform a second needle decompression on the same side. Successful needle decompression converts a tension pneumothorax into a simple pneumothorax. All of these patients will require a chest tube on arrival in the emergency department.

6. Place a finger from a surgical glove over the catheter hub. Cut a small hole in the end of the finger to make a one-way or flutter valve. Secure the glove finger to the catheter, using tape or a rubber band. The flutter valve collapses during inspiration and opens during expiration (Figure 3-23, *A* and *B*). In some EMS systems a Heimlich valve is used in place of the surgical glove finger.

7. Secure the catheter to the chest wall with a dressing and tape (Figure 3-24).

◆ Pulling It All Together

The management of circulatory (and ventilatory) emergencies must be performed efficiently and competently. A paramedic has a responsibility to the patient to stay up-to-date on current treatments and research, as well as to spend time practicing skills on mannequins or cadavers. To use an old phrase, "practice makes perfect!"

Testing Your Knowledge

1. List three methods for applying the pneumatic antishock garment.

2. All of the following are signs or symptoms of tension pneumothorax except:
   a. Bilateral distended neck veins
   b. Tracheal deviation toward the unaffected side
   c. Narrowing of the intercostal spaces on the affected side
   d. Respiratory distress or failure

3. When decompressing the chest of a patient with a suspected tension pneumothorax, it is important to insert the needle just over the top of the rib. This allows you to miss the blood vessels and nerves on the underside of the rib.
   a. True
   b. False

4. From the following list, select the situations in which the PASG is indicated.
   I. Suspected internal abdominal hemorrhage
   II. Open fracture of the femur with associated hemorrhage
   III. Unstable pelvic fracture with borderline hypotension
   IV. Left congestive heart failure with uncompensated hypotension

   Select your answer from the following:
   a. I and III
   b. II and IV
   c. I, II, and III
   d. II, III, and IV

5. Suspicion of tension pneumothorax would be based on all of the following signs/symptoms except:
   a. Distended jugular veins
   b. Displacement of the trachea away from the affected side
   c. Poor perfusion
   d. Hyporesonance over the suspected lung field

6. If thoracic decompression is performed on an uninjured chest, the result may be:
   a. Cardiac tamponade
   b. Aortic stenosis
   c. Simple pneumothorax
   d. Aortic puncture

7. From the following list of signs, select the one that is NOT considered an indication of possible IV infiltration?

    a. Swelling at the venipuncture site
    b. Inability to aspirate blood
    c. No flashback of blood in the tubing
    d. Progressively increasing drip rate

8. If possible, the paramedic should use which of the following IV catheter sizes when starting an IV in the shock patient?

    a. 16-gauge
    b. 18-gauge
    c. 20-gauge
    d. Largest bore possible

9. When initiating an IV using an over-the-needle catheter, the paramedic should never reinsert the needle through the catheter because of the danger of which of the following?

    a. Infiltration
    b. Contamination
    c. Trauma to the inside of the vein
    d. Causing a catheter embolus

10. From the following list, select a "trick of the trade" that can be used to help distend the jugular veins before venipuncture.

    a. Place pressure just above the clavicle.
    b. Elevate the patient's legs.
    c. Tap the neck area in order to agitate the vessel.
    d. a and b

11. Five minutes after initiating an IV in the hand of a 74-year-old patient experiencing severe pulmonary edema, you note that the area seems swollen and the intravenous drip has stopped. You have a 15-minute estimated time of arrival at the hospital. You should immediately discontinue the IV, remove the catheter, and reinitiate it in the other arm.

    a. True
    b. False

12. The external jugular vein is considered a peripheral IV site.

    a. True
    b. False

Answers are in Appendix A.

BIBLIOGRAPHY

Bickell WH, Pepe PE, Bailey ML, et al: Randomized trial of pneumatic antishock garments in the prehospital management of penetrating abdominal injuries, *Ann Emerg Med* 16:653-658, 1987.

Caroline NL: *Emergency care in the streets*, ed 3, Boston, 1987, Little, Brown, pp 83-94, 89-93, 204-206.

Cosentino F, Vail P, Rose M: Performing basic IV procedures. In West RS, editor: *Managing IV therapy*, Horsham, Pa, 1981, Intermed Communications, pp 24-48.

Fowler RL: Shock. In Campbell JE, editor: *Basic trauma life support: advanced prehospital care*, ed 2, Englewood Cliffs, NJ, 1988, Prentice-Hall, pp 361-371.

Jorden RC: Shock. In Tintinalli JE, Krome RL, Ruiz E, editors: *Emergency medicine: a comprehensive study guide*, ed 2, New York, 1988, McGraw-Hill, pp 109-117.

Mannix KL: Hemorrhagic shock. In Rosen P, Baker II FJ, Barkin RM, et al, editors: *Emergency medicine: concepts and clinical practice*, ed 2, vol 1, St Louis, 1988, Mosby, pp 179-202.

Mattox KL, Bickell W, Pepe PE, et al: Prospective MAST study in 911 patients, *J Trauma* 29:1104-1112, 1989.

Mattox KL, Bickell WH, Pepe PE, et al: Prospective randomized evaluation of antishock MAST in post-traumatic hypotension, *J Trauma* 26:779-786, 1986.

McSwain NE Jr: Pneumatic antishock garment: state of the art 1988, *Ann Emerg Med* 17:506-525, 1988.

Norton R, Frumkin K: The pneumatic antishock garment. In Roberts JR, Hedges JR, editors: *Clinical procedures in emergency medicine*, ed 2, Philadelphia, 1991, WB Saunders, 1991, pp 421-431.

Ross DS: Thoracentesis. In Roberts JR, Hedges JR, editors: *Clinical procedures in emergency medicine*, ed 2, Philadelphia, 1991, WB Saunders, 1991, pp 112-128.

Simon RR, Brenner BE: *Procedures and techniques in emergency medicine*, ed 2, Baltimore, 1987, Williams and Wilkins, pp 361-362.

Subcommittee on ATLS, Committee on Trauma of the American College of Surgeons: *Advanced trauma life support instructor manual*, Chicago, 1989, American College of Surgeons, pp 68-69.

Tintinalli JE, Ravikrishman KP: Spontaneous and iatrogenic pneumothorax. In Tintinalli JE, Krome RL, Ruiz E, editors: *Emergency medicine: a comprehensive study guide*, ed 2, New York, New York, 1988, McGraw-Hill, pp 269-271.

Vukich DJ, Markovchick VJ: Pulmonary and chest wall injuries. In Rosen P, Baker FJ II, Barkin RM, et al, editors: *Emergency medicine: concepts and clinical practice*, ed 2, vol 1, St Louis, 1988, Mosby, pp 473-486.

Wyte SR, Barker WJ: Central venous catheterization: Internal jugular approach and alternatives. In Roberts JR, Hodges JR, editors: *Clinical procedures in emergency medicine*, ed 2, Philadelphia, 1991, WB Saunders, pp 340-351.

Pneumatic Antishock Garment

This skill section is divided into two parts; application and inflation, and deflation and removal. The paramedic should be able to complete both sections in 8 minutes. (This is strictly a PASG skill station; patient assessment is evaluated separately).

Pneumatic Antishock Garment	Possible points	Points awarded
Application and inflation:		
Evaluate vital signs.	1	
Prepare garment and place next to patient.	1	
Place patient onto garment (supine).	1	
Ensure that top of garment is just inferior to twelfth rib.	1	
Wrap each section of garment around respective area and secure velcro.	3	
Attach foot pump.	1	
Open appropriate stopcock valve(s).	1	
Inflate garment using foot pump.	1	
Close stopcock valves.	1	
Reevaluate vital signs.	1	
(If using sectional inflation procedure, repeat above four steps until garment is completely inflated.		
Deflation and removal:		
Reevaluate vital signs.	1	
Ensure that all stopcocks are closed.	1	
Disconnect rubber hose stopcocks.	1	
Open abdominal stopcock and allow for release of air for 4 to 5 seconds.	1	
Reevaluate vital signs.	1	
Repeat abdominal deflation until completely deflated.	1	
Open leg stopcock and allow for release of air for 4 to 5 seconds (1 point per leg).	2	
Reevaluate vital signs.	1	
Repeat leg deflation until both legs are completely deflated (1 point per leg).	2	
SUBTOTAL FROM APPLICATION/INFLATION	**12**	
SUBTOTAL FROM DEFLATION/REMOVAL	**11**	
TOTAL SCORE	**23**	

COMMENTS _____

_____

_____

Peripheral Intravenous Therapy

This skill should take no longer than 6 minutes to complete.

Procedure	Possible points	Points awarded
Assemble necessary equipment, selecting proper solution and administration set for given scenario.	2	
Check solution and date.	1	
Prepare solution and set, including flushing the tubing of air. Prepare strips of tape.	2	
Observe universal precautions.	1	
Apply tourniquet.	1	
Locate suitable vein.	1	
Cleanse venipuncture site.	1	
Correctly perform venipuncture.	1	
Note blood return.	1	
Advance catheter and remove needle.	1	
Release tourniquet.	1	
Connect IV tubing.	1	
Adjust flow rate.	1	
Apply povidone-iodine ointment and tape securely.	1	
Use aseptic technique throughout procedure.	1	
Dispose of needle properly.	1	
TOTAL SCORE	**18**	

COMMENTS _____

_____

_____

External Jugular Vein Cannulation

This skill should take no longer than 6 minutes to complete.

Procedure	Possible points	Points awarded
Assemble necessary equipment, selecting proper solution and administration set for given scenario.	2	
Check solution and date.	1	
Prepare solution and set, including flushing the tubing of air. Prepare strips of tape.	2	
Observe universal precautions.	1	
Place patient supine and elevate legs. Locate suitable vein.	2	
Cleanse venipuncture site.	1	
Pull tension on vein just above angle of jaw and correctly perform venipuncture.	1	
Note blood return.	1	
Advance catheter and remove needle.	1	
Connect IV tubing.	1	
Adjust flow rate.	1	
Apply povidone-iodine ointment and tape securely.	1	
Use aseptic technique throughout procedure.	1	
TOTAL SCORE	16	

COMMENTS _____

_____

_____

Thoracic Decompression

Thoracic decompression is the procedure of placing a large-bore catheter through the chest wall and into the pleural cavity. The use of a 14-gauge (or larger) catheter is a quick method of providing temporary relief to the patient experiencing tension pneumothorax. This skill should take no longer than 6 minutes to complete.

Procedure	Possible points	Points awarded
Observe universal precautions.	1	
Evaluate chest to verify absence of breath sounds.	1	
Assemble equipment.	1	
Cleanse chest wall in preparation for puncture.	1	
Attach syringe to catheter and insert into chest at appropriate site.	2	
Appreciate "pop" and listen for escape of air (or immediate movement of plunger up the barrel of the syringe).	1	
Advance catheter and remove needle.	1	
Place finger from surgical glove over catheter hub. Cut small hole in end of finger to make flutter valve. Secure with tape or rubber band.	2	
Secure catheter and glove to chest wall using appropriate method.	1	
TOTAL	**11**	

COMMENTS _____

_____

_____

CHAPTER FOUR

Medication Administration

Objectives

A paramedic should be able to—

1. State the definition of subcutaneous injection.

2. List two examples of medical conditions in which subcutaneous injection of epinephrine may be lifesaving.

3. List the indications for subcutaneous injection.

4. List the steps involved in the technique of subcutaneous injection.

5. State the definition of intramuscular injection.

6. List one indication for giving an intramuscular injection in the prehospital setting.

7. List three medications that may be administered intramuscularly in the prehospital setting.

8. Demonstrate giving an intramuscular injection on a simulation mannequin.

9. State the definition of intravenous bolus.

10. List two indications when intravenous bolus is the preferred route of medication administration.

11. List six emergencies in which intravenous bolus is commonly used.

12. Demonstrate giving an intravenous bolus on a simulation mannequin.

13. State the definition of intravenous drip infusion.

14. Given a simulation mannequin, demonstrate the procedure for setting up and administering an intravenous drip infusion.

15. State the definition of endotracheal bolus.

16. State when endotracheal bolus is more advantageous than traditional routes of medication administration.

17. List the five medications that may be administered via an endotracheal tube (ETT).

18. Explain why CPR must be momentarily stopped when administering a medication via an ETT.

19. State the definition of intravenous drip infusion.

20. List two indications for intravenous drip infusion.

21. List the steps involved in the technique of intravenous infusion.

22. State the definition of nebulized inhalation of medication.

23. List the main indication for administering a drug by nebulizer.

24. List two common inhaled bronchodilators used for nebulized inhalation.

25. List the equipment required for nebulized inhalation.

26. Demonstrate the procedure involved for providing nebulized inhalation to a patient.

27. State the definition of self-administered nitrous oxide.

28. List the percentages of oxygen and nitrous oxide in Nitronox.

29. List the effects of nitrous oxide on the following:
    a. Central nervous system
    b. Respiratory system
    c. Cough and gag reflex

30. List three indications for use of nitrous oxide.

31. List six contraindications for nitrous oxide.

32. List the steps involved in the technique of nitrous oxide administration.

33. Differentiate between an indwelling and an implantable catheter.

Photo courtesy Colin Williams.

Case Scenario

You are dispatched to the "Pirate's Inn," which is a seafood restaurant in your oceanside community, for a "patient who can't breathe."

The patient is a 55-year-old male who appears to be in anaphylaxis secondary to iodine allergy (from the seafood). His wife tells you that he is aware of his allergy, but always takes an antihistamine tablet before he eats shrimp. "He's done this many times before and has never had a reaction 'this bad.'" He has no other pertinent medical history to report.

The patient is moved to the stretcher and evaluated. Physical examination notes an obese man who is in obvious respiratory distress. He has audible stridor. Speaking appears to be difficult. His skin is flushed, and he has a decreased level of consciousness. His blood pressure is 78/40; pulse is 134 and thready; and respiratory rate is 30 and

very labored, though little air seems to be moving into the lungs. Audible wheezes can be heard. EKG is sinus tachycardia.

While assessing the patient, you initiate oxygen therapy at 15 L/ minute via nonrebreather mask. Venous status seems poor; thus you administer epinephrine 0.03 mg 1:1000 subcutaneously in the left arm while an intravenous line (IV) site is located. After 3 minutes, BP is 82/42, pulse is 138, and respirations are 30 and still labored. You initiate an IV of lactated Ringer's in the right antecubital vein, using a 16-gauge catheter. You consult Medical Control and request epinephrine 0.05 mg 1:10,000 intravenous bolus. The physician is particularly concerned about the patient's airway because of laryngeal edema. Intubation is recommended if the patient fails to improve rapidly.

Five minutes after the epinephrine 1:10,000 bolus, the patient's respiratory distress greatly im-

proves, and air is once again moving into his lungs. Mentation and color improve dramatically. Blood pressure is 104/76, pulse is 106, and respirations are 24 and move with ease.

You transport the patient to the Medical Center for follow-up evaluation and care. Following testing and education about the hazards of self-medication and allergic reactions, the patient is released to the care of his wife.

This section reviews the more traditional medication routes, along with those newer to the prehospital field. Subcutaneous injection, intramuscular injection, intravenous drip infusion, intravenous bolus, endotracheal bolus, nebulized inhalation, self-administered nitrous oxide with oxygen, and alternate intravenous medication routes are discussed. Routes specific to the pediatric patient, such as intraosseous infusion, are discussed in Chapter 6.

◆ Subcutaneous Injection

Subcutaneous (SQ) injection is a method of administering drugs directly into subcutaneous or fatty tissue where they are absorbed into the general circulation.

Background

Subcutaneous injection is one of the simpler forms of drug administration that indeed may be lifesaving in cases of severe asthma or allergic reactions in which epinephrine 1:1000 is required. Some emergency medical service (EMS) systems carry glucagon for insulin shock, which may be administered subcutaneously when other routes are not easily available. It is important to ensure that the subcutaneous injection is an administration of drug into the subcutaneous tissue rather than into the more superficial dermis or deeper muscle, connective tissue or blood vessels. Medication injected subcutaneously is

typically absorbed more slowly than the intravenous or intramuscular routes, but faster than the oral route.

Indications

Subcutaneous injection is indicated for administration of a limited number of drugs in specific clinical settings, commonly asthma and allergic/anaphylactic reactions.

Contraindications

There are no contraindications to subcutaneous infusion, except for medications not delivered by that route.

Equipment (Figure 4-1)

◆ 25-gauge, ½-inch needle
◆ Tuberculin 1-cc syringe
◆ Povidone-iodine or alcohol preps
◆ Gloves
◆ 2×2-inch sterile gauze pads
◆ Sharps container

Procedure

1. Observe universal precautions (gloves).
2. Confirm the drug order, amount to be given, and route.

PEARLS & PITFALLS

Things to Watch Out For...

Since small volumes (1 to 2 cc) of drug are usually used in subcutaneous injections, be careful in pulling up the exact amount into the syringe. In prefilled syringes, wasting the excess before administration allows for the exact dosage to be given.

Note that a poor patient response to a medication could mean that you have inadvertently injected the dermis instead of the subcutaneous tissue.

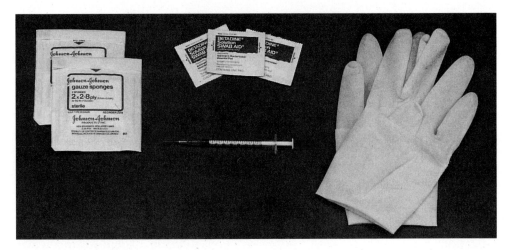

Figure 4-1 Equipment for subcutaneous injection: 25-gauge ½-inch needle, 1-cc syringe, preps, gloves.

3. Explain the procedure to the patient and reconfirm that the patient is not allergic to the medication.

4. Check the medication name, expiration, coloration, and clarity.

5. Assemble the equipment and attach the needle to the syringe if not preattached.

6. Calculate and draw up the desired volume of drug into the syringe.

7. Eject any air from the syringe.

8. Identify an injection site—the area over the deltoid muscle of the shoulder is commonly used.

9. Clean the injection site with alcohol or povidone iodine (Figure 4-2).

10. Apply tension to (or tent) the skin to pull it away from underlying muscle.

11. Advise the patient to expect a stick.

12. Insert the needle at a 45-degree angle into the subcutaneous tissue.

13. Pull back, or aspirate, on the syringe (Figure 4-3). If a blood vessel has been entered, you will see blood return in the syringe (Figure 4-4). In the event that this occurs, remove the needle and begin again, using a different site. Apply pressure over the site with a sterile gauze pad. If performed correctly, air bubbles may appear in the syringe.

14. Inject the drug into the subcutaneous tissue slowly.

15. Withdraw the needle and apply pressure to the site with a sterile gauze pad.

16. Properly dispose of the syringe and medication container.

17. Monitor the patient for medication effect.

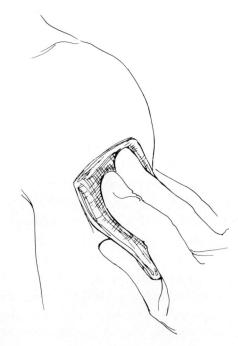

Figure 4-2 Cleanse injection site with alcohol or povidone-iodine.

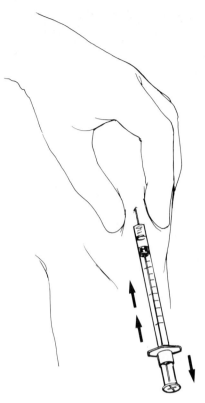

Absorption Problems

Poor perfusion can result in delayed absorption of subcutaneous or intramuscular injected medications. In addition, cold ambient temperature slows absorption, whereas warm ambient temperature hastens absorption.

Figure 4-3 Insert needle into subcutaneous tissue and pull back on the syringe.

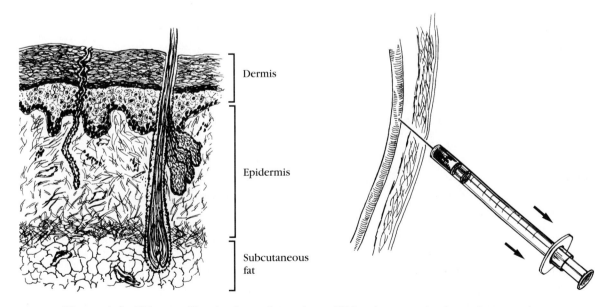

Dermis

Epidermis

Subcutaneous fat

Figure 4-4 When pulling back on the syringe, if blood returns in the syringe, you've entered a blood vessel. Withdraw the needle and start over.

◆ Intramuscular Injection

Intramuscular (IM) injection is a method of administering drugs directly into muscle, where they are subsequently absorbed into the general circulation.

Background

The administration of intramuscular drugs in the field is relatively uncommon. Prehospital drugs that may be administered intramuscularly include, but are not limited to, diazepam, meperidine, morphine, and glucagon. This method is particularly useful when other administration routes fail. Compared with intravenous injection, absorption via the intramuscular route is slower and requires adequate perfusion. For example, the intramuscular route may be ineffective when the patient is hypotensive.

Indications

Intramuscular injection is indicated for the administration of specific drugs in the prehospital setting when slow absorption is acceptable, or when other administration routes are unsuccessful.

Contraindications

Intramuscular injections may be contraindicated in patients with coagulopathies (a defect in the clotting mechanism of the body) or those who take anticoagulants.

Equipment

* 21-gauge needle
* Syringe
* Povidone-iodine or alcohol preps
* Gloves
* Sharps container

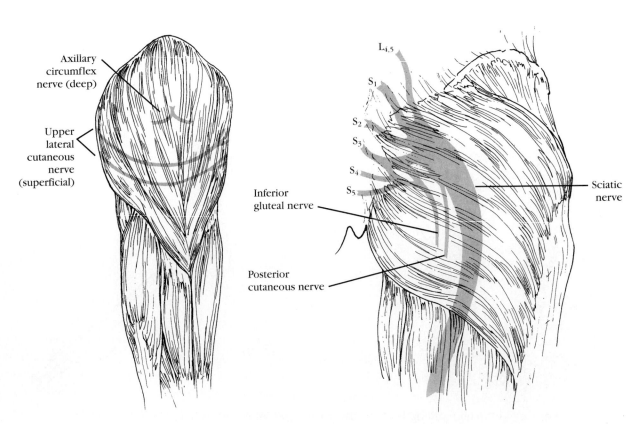

Figure 4-5 Anatomy of the deltoid and gluteal areas.

Procedure

1. Observe universal precautions (gloves).

2. Confirm the drug order, amount to be given, and route.

3. Explain the procedure to the patient and reconfirm that the patient is not allergic to the medication.

4. Check the medication name, expiration, coloration, and clarity.

5. Assemble equipment and attach the needle to the syringe if not preattached.

6. Calculate and draw up the desired volume of drug into the syringe.

7. Eject any air from the syringe.

8. Identify an injection site. The deltoid muscle of the shoulder and upper arm and the upper outside quadrant of the gluteus muscle are commonly used sites (Figure 4-5).

9. Cleanse the injection site with alcohol or povidone-iodine.

10. Stretch or "flatten" the skin overlying the site with your fingers.

11. Advise the patient to expect a stick.

12. Insert the needle at a 90-degree angle (Figure 4-6).

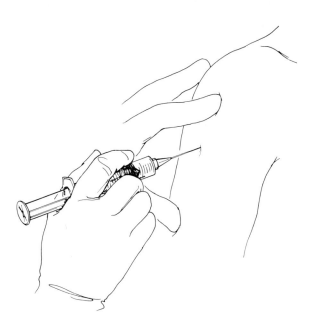

Figure 4-6 Insert needle at 90-degree angle.

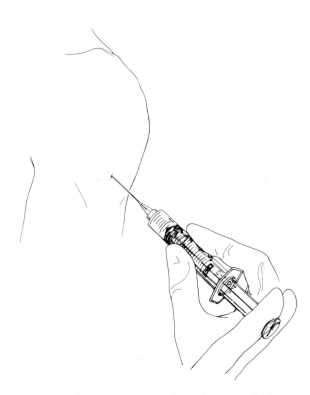

Figure 4-7 Aspirate, looking for air bubbles.

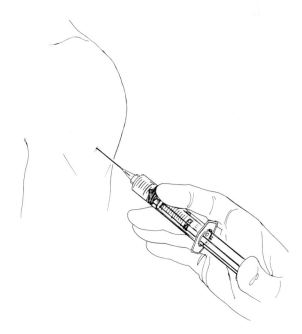

Figure 4-8 Slowly inject the medication into the muscle.

13. Pull back, or aspirate, on the syringe (Figure 4-7). If a blood vessel has been entered, you will see blood return in the syringe. If this happens, withdraw the needle, apply direct pressure with a sterile gauze pad, and prepare to restick the patient with a new needle.

14. Inject the drug into the muscle slowly (Figure 4-8).

15. Withdraw the needle and apply pressure to the site with a sterile gauze pad or iodine/alcohol prep.

16. Properly dispose of the syringe and medication container.

17. Monitor the patient for medication effect.

PEARLS
&
PITFALLS

Giving an Injection That Doesn't Hurt...

Most patients have high anxiety on hearing the word "needle." Several things can be done so that the IM injection does not cause undo pain to your patient. Try these tips the next time you give an injection.

- Always allow the alcohol or iodine solution to dry before puncturing the skin. Wet solution will often adhere to the needle and result in a burning sensation to the patient.
- Tell the patient that the injection will probably hurt for a few moments, rather than just saying that "there's going to be a little stick." Most patients appreciate your honesty.
- A slow, steady administration is less traumatic than a rapid, pushing motion on the syringe.
- Be sure that you have inserted the needle far enough to penetrate the appropriate layer of skin.

♦ Intravenous Bolus

Intravenous bolus, or "IV push," is a method of administering drugs directly into the vein. This method of administration allows for a rapid onset of medications, especially in critical situations.

Background

As the most rapid method of drug administration available to paramedics, intravenous bolus is most commonly used for life-threatening emergencies and cardiopulmonary arrest. These emergencies include, but are not limited to:

- Ventricular dysrhythmias
- Supraventricular tachycardia
- Symptomatic bradycardia
- Hypoglycemia
- Metabolic acidosis
- Seizures
- Acute pulmonary edema
- Cardiopulmonary arrest
- Narcotic overdose
- Pain control

Because of the emergent nature of these conditions, many of these drugs come in commonly used dosages in prefilled syringes for convenience and ease of administration.

Indications

Intravenous bolus drug administration is indicated for the rapid delivery of drugs.

Contraindications

Intravenous bolus drug administration may be ineffective at sites in close proximity to dialysis shunts or traumatized areas.

Equipment

- Appropriate size syringe and needle for amount of medication to be delivered (or medication in prefilled syringe) (Figures 4-9 and 4-10)
- Appropriate medication
- Alcohol preps

◆ Gloves
◆ Sharps container

Procedure

This procedure assumes that an IV has previously been established and that a prefilled syringe is being used.

1. Observe universal precautions (gloves).

2. Confirm the drug order, amount to be given, and route.

3. Explain the procedure to the patient and reconfirm that the patient is not allergic to the medication.

4. Check the medication name, expiration, coloration, and clarity.

5. Assemble the appropriate equipment.

6. Calculate the desired volume of drug. If the entire syringe is not going to be given, the paramedic can either carefully inject the appropriate amount of drug or squirt out the excess amount.

7. Eject any air from the syringe.

8. Cleanse the rubber injection port with an alcohol prep (Figure 4-11).

9. Insert the needle into the rubber injection port.

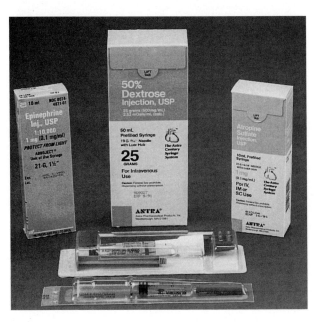

Figure 4-9 Packaged prefilled medications.

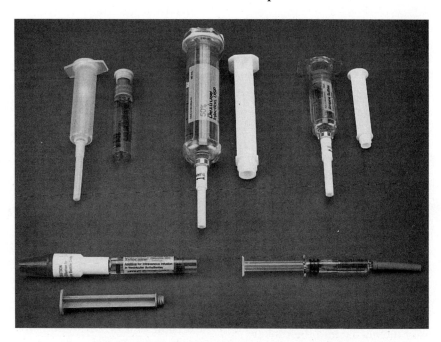

Figure 4-10 Medications in prefilled syringes.

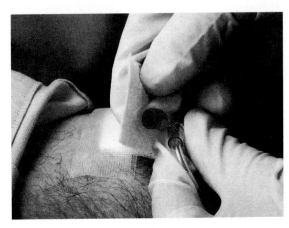

Figure 4-11 Wipe off the rubber injection port with alcohol.

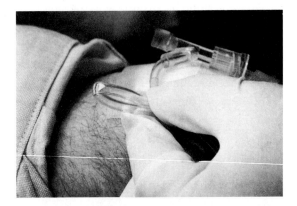

Figure 4-12 Pinch off IV tubing just above the injection port.

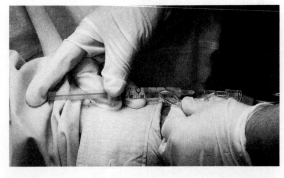

Figure 4-13 Insert the needle into the rubber injection port and slowly inject the desired amount of medication.

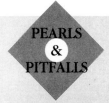

PEARLS & PITFALLS

IV Bolus Tips

Even though the needle used during an intravenous bolus does not come in direct contact with the patient, precaution is still advised. It is very easy to stick yourself while trying to insert a needle into an injection port, especially when trying to administer a medication in the back of a moving ambulance.

Always be sure that the IV is patent before injecting any medication by pulling back, or aspirating, on the plunger of the syringe. Resistance probably indicates a poorly positioned or infiltrated IV site. Medications such as 50% dextrose and norepinephrine may result in severe tissue necrosis.

10. Pinch off the IV tubing just above the injection port (Figure 4-12).

11. Inject the desired amount of medication into the injection port. Speed of administration is based on the individual drug (Figure 4-13).

12. Release or unpinch the IV tubing.

13. Flush the IV tubing. Run enough fluid in (no greater than 20 cc) to ensure delivery of drug through the tubing into the circulation.

14. Readjust the IV flow to the previous rate.

15. Properly dispose of the syringe and medication container.

16. Monitor the patient for medication effect.

◆ Intravenous Drip Infusion (Intravenous Piggyback)

Intravenous drip infusion or IV piggyback (IVPB) provides a route for continuous administration of a medication. This is accomplished by connecting an IV infusion containing a medication to a preexisting IV site.

IV Fluid and Drug Calculations

Barry Bunn, EMT-P

There are many ways to make medication administration and IV drip rate problems easy to remember. This section provides a summary of easy formulas for the prehospital provider.

Flow rate calculations

$$gtt/min = \frac{\text{Volume to be infused} \times \text{gtt/ml of solution set}}{\text{Total time of infusion in minutes}}$$

Practice problem

A physician orders you to hang an IV for a GI bleed patient. He orders NaCL at 300 ml/hr. You have a macro-drip solution set.

Solution:

$$\frac{300 \text{ ml} \times 10 \text{ gtt/ml}}{60 \text{ min/hour}} = 50 \text{ gtt/min}$$

Simple drug dosage calculations
Definitions

1. Want—what the physician orders
2. Vehicle—what volume the medication is packaged
3. Have—the packaged amount of the medication

ml to
be given =

$$\frac{\text{Amount ordered}}{\text{Concentration available}} = \frac{\text{want} \times \text{Vehicle}}{\text{have}}$$

Practice problem

A physician orders 60 mg of furosemide intravenously. You have furosemide, 20 mg/2 ml. How many milliliters would you give?

Solution

$$\frac{60 \text{ mg} \times 2 \text{ ml}}{20 \text{ mg}} = 6 \text{ ml}$$

Complex drug dosage calculation

$$\text{Desired rate (gtt/min)} = \frac{\text{Dose } (\mu g/kg) \times \text{Patient's weight (kg)} \times 60 \,(gtt/ml)}{\text{Concentration on hand} \times \text{time}}$$

Practice problem

The physician asks you to add 200 mg of dopamine to a 250-ml bag of D_5W and infuse it at 2 μg/kg/min. Your patient weighs 220 lb. How many gtt/min will you infuse?

Solution

Step 1: Convert patient's weight to kilograms
   1 lb = 2.2 kg/lb: therefore 220 lb ÷ 2.2 kg/lb
   = 100 kg

Step 2: Convert milligrams of dopamine to micrograms of dopamine
   1 mg = 1000 μg
   200 mg × 1000 μg/mg = 200,000

Step 3: Calculate how much dopamine you have per milliliter of intravenous fluid.
   200,000 μg in 250 ml of D_5W
   200,000 μg/250 ml = 800 μg/ml

Step 4: Plug in your values

$$\frac{2 \,\mu g/kg \times 100 \text{ kg} \times 60 \text{ gtt/ml}}{800 \,\mu g/ml \times 1 \text{ minute}} = 15 \text{ gtt/min}$$

Remember

- If you put 200 mg in 250 ml, it yields 800 μg/ml.
- If you put 400 mg in 250 ml, it yields 1600 μg/ml.
- If you put 800 mg in 250 ml, it yields 3200 μg/ml.
- If you stock 500 ml of D_5W, double the amount of dopamine to give the same concentrations.

Background

Intravenous drip infusion is a continuous method of medication administration. It offers the advantage of being easily titrated to increase or decrease the rate of flow or to discontinue the infusion, depending on the patient's response. The correct computation of the amount of medication to be added to the intravenous solution and the rate at which it should be delivered are most important.

Indications

Intravenous drip infusion is indicated for drugs that require continuous infusion and/or titration of dose.

Contraindications

Intravenous drip infusion may be ineffective at sites in close proximity to dialysis shunts or traumatized areas.

Equipment

- Intravenous solution to which the medication will be added, usually 5% dextrose.
- Mini-drip (micro) IV tubing
- 19-gauge needle
- Alcohol preps
- Gloves
- Syringe and needle
- 1-inch tape
- Medication label

Procedure

This procedure assumes that an IV has already been established (Figures 4-14 and 4-15).

1. Observe universal precautions (gloves).

2. Confirm the drug order, amount to be given, and route.

3. Explain the procedure to the patient and reconfirm that the patient is not allergic to the medication.

4. Check the medication name, expiration, coloration, and clarity.

5. Assemble the equipment and attach the needle to the syringe if not preattached.

6. Calculate and draw up the desired volume of drug into the syringe.

7. Check the intravenous fluid for proper fluid, expiration date, and clarity.

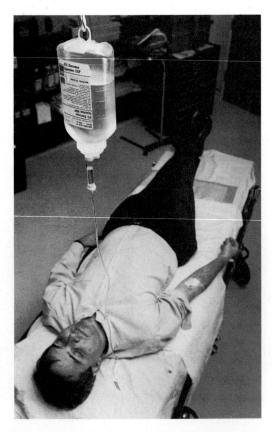

Figure 4-14   IV already established in patient.

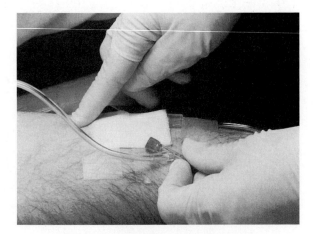

Figure 4-15   Isolate injection port.

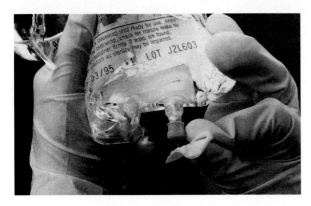

Figure 4-16 Cleanse the injection port of the IV bag or bottle with an alcohol prep.

8. Cleanse the injection port on the IV bag or bottle with an alcohol prep (Figure 4-16).

9. Insert the needle into the injection port on the IV bag or bottle and inject the volume of the drug ordered (Figure 4-17).

10. Mix the drug in the intravenous solution by gently shaking the bag (Figure 4-18).

11. Using a medication label, identify the bag with the time, amount injected, concentration of medication in the fluid, and your initials (Figure 4-19).

12. Attach the administration set and purge the line of air. This will provide you with a line filled with medication. A micro-drip set should be used with prehospital IVPBs.

13. Attach a sterile needle to the administration set. Clean the injection port nearest to the patient and attach the IVPB to this site.

14. Set the primary IV rate to KVO.

15. Calculate the rate of administration to achieve the desired dose and adjust the flow rate accordingly (Figure 4-20).

16. Secure the IVPB with tape to prevent accidental dislodgement of the needle.

17. Monitor the patient for medication effect.

◆ Endotracheal Bolus

Endotracheal bolus is a procedure that allows the delivery of a medication directly to the tracheobronchial tree and lung tissue, via an ETT.

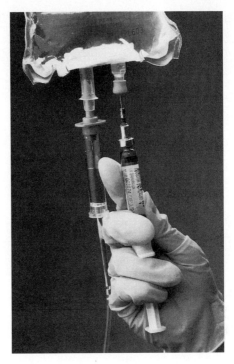

Figure 4-17 Insert the needle into the port and inject the appropriate amount of medication into the IV bag or bottle.

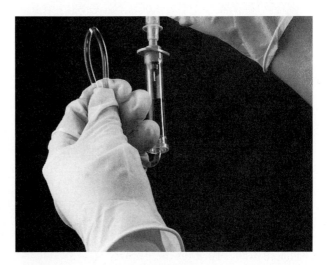

Figure 4-18 Mix the drug with the intravenous solution by gently shaking.

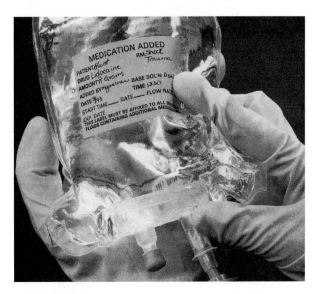

Figure 4-19   Label the solution with the time, amount injected, concentration of the medication in the fluid, and your initials.

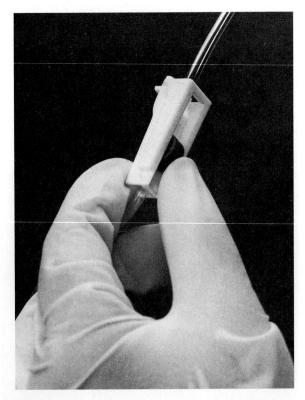

Figure 4-20   Turn off the primary KVO IV line. Adjust the flow rate to deliver the desired amount of medication.

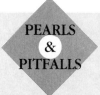

PEARLS
&
PITFALLS

Piggyback Problems

As with intravenous boluses, it is very easy to stick yourself with the needle while trying to insert it into the injection port. Be careful, especially if you are in the back of a moving ambulance.

Always make sure that your medications are compatible. In most cases, after initiating an IVPB in one arm, you should immediately start another IV in the other arm, just for intravenous boluses. Labeling is important. Without an identifying label, most IVs and medications look the same.

Background

Administration of medication via an ETT is generally reserved for use during cardiac arrest or when intravenous access is not available. The number of drugs that may be given via an ETT is limited. Paramedics most often administer three drugs during cardiopulmonary arrest: atropine, epinephrine, and lidocaine. Two other medications can be given when necessary via ETT: naloxone (Narcan) and diazepam (Valium). Hence, the mnemonic "NAVEL" was developed, which stands for Narcan (naloxone), atropine, Valium, epinephrine, and lidocaine, respectively. The exact dose of drug administered via this route is still under investigation, but for now the ET dose of a drug should be at least equal to the intravenous dose and should be delivered in a volume of 5 to 10 ml.

Indications

Endotracheal bolus drug administration is indicated for certain drugs during cardiopulmonary arrest or when intravenous access is not available.

PEARLS
&
PITFALLS

Another Way To Do It...

There is more than one way to accomplish a goal. The following technique is used in some EMS systems, instead of constantly removing the bag to administer the drug down the tube.

- Place a needle or IV catheter through the side of the ETT so that it protrudes into the tube lumen. The medication can then be injected via needle if you are using regular syringes instead of prefills.

- This technique offers the advantage that no interruption of ventilation occurs and the drug is forced into the tracheo-bronchial tree (Figure 4-21, *A* and *B*).

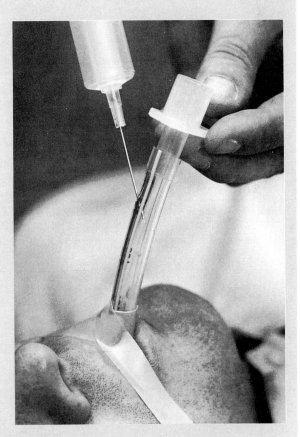

B

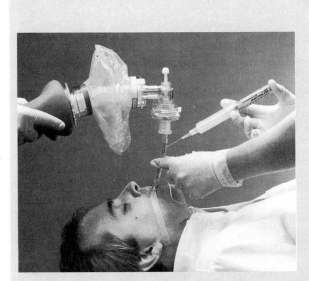

A

Figure 4-21   A and **B**, An alternate method is to place a needle through the side of the ETT. This allows you to inject medication without stopping ventilations.

PEARLS & PITFALLS

Oops!

Generally speaking, it only takes making an error once to remember **NOT** to do something again. Such is the case when giving a medication via ETT during cardiac arrest. Cardiopulmonary resuscitation (CPR) must be terminated when pushing the medication via ETT, or all the medication will be blown back out of the tube as a result of chest compression. Quickly administer the bolus, hyperventilate for 10 seconds, then reinitiate chest compressions. This will allow for the drug to diffuse across the alveolar membranes.

Contraindications

There are no specific contraindications to administering drugs via an ETT. However, the paramedic must remember the five medications listed above that can be given via ETT without detriment to the patient.

Equipment

- Prefilled syringe and needle or 18- or 19-gauge needle with syringe
- Sterile saline or water, if the medication needs to be diluted
- Sharps container

Procedure

The following procedure outlines the method used for administering a medication that comes in a prefilled syringe. It is taken for granted that this patient is already intubated (Figure 4-22).

1. Observe universal precautions (gloves).
2. Confirm the drug order, amount to be given, and route.

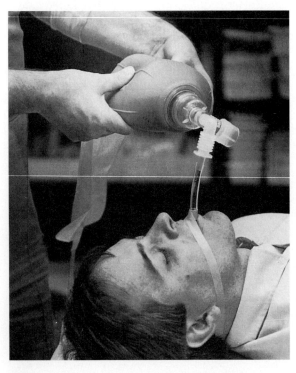

Figure 4-22 Patient with a properly secured ETT in place.

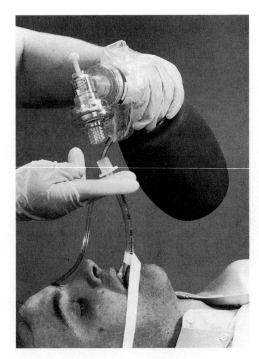

Figure 4-23 Disconnect the bag-valve device from the ETT.

3. Check the medication name, expiration, coloration, and clarity.

4. Assemble the syringe.

5. Calculate the desired volume of drug. If the entire syringe is not going to be given, the paramedic can either carefully inject the appropriate amount of drug or squirt out the excess amount.

6. Hyperventilate the patient per ETT.

7. Disconnect the ETT from the bag-valve device (Figure 4-23).

8. Stop chest compressions.

9. Place the needle into the lumen of the ETT and forcefully inject the solution (Figure 4-24).

10. Reconnect the bag-valve device (Figure 4-25) and hyperventilate the patient for 10 seconds to facilitate drug delivery farther into the tracheobronchial tree.

11. Resume appropriate ventilation and reverify ETT placement. Also reinitiate chest compressions.

12. Verify the placement of the ETT. It is not uncommon for the tube to be displaced from the trachea and accidently repositioned in the esophagus during this procedure.

13. Monitor the patient for medication effect.

◆ Nebulized Inhalation

Nebulized inhalation of drugs is a method of delivering medications via the tracheobronchial tree, using a device known as a nebulizer. This process mixes high-flow oxygen and a medication, which results in a vapor that the patient can inhale.

Background

Paramedics frequently see patients with hand-held nebulizers. Many EMS systems have incorporated nebulized drug administration into their treatment regimens for asthma and

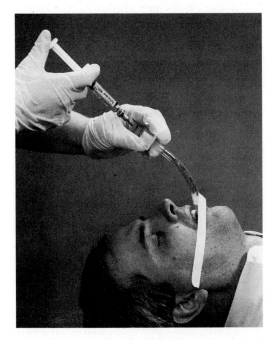

Figure 4-24 Forcefully inject the drug into the lumen of the ETT.

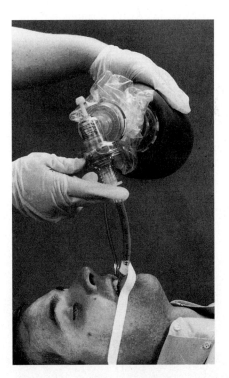

Figure 4-25 Reconnect the bag-valve device to the ETT, using care not to accidentally dislodge the tube from the trachea. Hyperventilate the patient for up to 10 seconds or give five rapid insufflations to facilitate the drug delivery to the alveoli.

chronic obstructive pulmonary disease (COPD). Inhaled bronchodilators, such as albuterol (Proventil) and metaproterenol (Alupent), are commonly used in hand-held and side-stream nebulizers. Most prehospital medications are given via side-stream devices, which mix oxygen with the medication. Some attachments also allow a nebulized mist to be forced into a patient, using a bag-valve-mask when the patient is unable to adequately ventilate himself.

Indications

Nebulized inhalation is indicated for patients with asthma or COPD, who are in need of rapid bronchodilation.

Contraindications

The procedure of nebulized inhalation is not contraindicated for any patient. Specific contraindications are reserved to the medication (bronchodilator) to be inhaled by the patient.

Equipment

Side-stream nebulizer, which is driven with oxygen (Figure 4-26)
* Medication to be administered
* 0.3 cc of normal saline for dilution of the bronchodilator

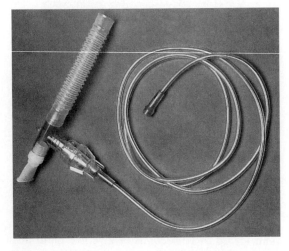

Figure 4-26 Side-stream nebulizer with oxygen tubing attached.

Procedure

1. Observe universal precautions (gloves are a minimum; mask and goggles are recommended since patients often experience violent coughing during treatments).

2. Explain the procedure to the patient.

3. Take the patient's vital signs and connect the patient to a cardiac monitor.

4. Assemble the nebulizer device. Place the bronchodilator and saline solution in the reservoir well of the side-stream nebulizer.

5. Connect the device and administer oxygen at 6 to 12 L/minute (according to the specific device) to start nebulizer treatment.

6. Have patient inhale normally through mouthpiece of nebulizer. The aerosol inhalation should start at the end of one tidal breath just as the patient initiates the next breath. The

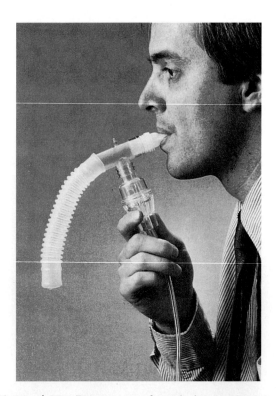

Figure 4-27 Proper use of a nebulizer containing a bronchodilation medication. The medication is placed in the small chamber just above this patient's hand. A bag-valve mask can be attached to the corrugated tubing to assist the patient with ventilation.

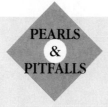

Side Effects

Bronchodilators may cause tachycardia and other dysrhythmias. All patients receiving these medications should be connected to a cardiac monitor. Treatment should be discontinued when cardiac side effects occur or when symptoms of breathing difficulty disappear.

inhalation should continue until the patient fully expands his or her lungs (Figure 4-27).

7. Have the patient take a deep breath every 3 to 5 inhalations.

8. The treatment should last until the solution is depleted.

9. Place the patient back onto supplemental oxygen following medication administration.

10. Monitor the patient, EKG, and vital signs for medication effect. Treatment should be discontinued if tachycardia greater than 120 beats per minute, ventricular ectopy, or paradoxic bronchospasm is noted.

♦ Self-Administered Nitrous Oxide (Nitronox)

A 50:50 nitrous and oxygen mixture, known as Nitronox, allows the patient to regulate his pain control by self-administering this gas, commonly known as "laughing gas."

Background

Inhalation of a preset 50:50 mixture of oxygen and nitrous oxide through self-administration is an important method of pain management in the prehospital setting. It can exert analgesic effects equivalent to 10 to 20

mg of intravenous morphine, without the side effects. Approximately 10% of patients are "nonresponders" to the gas. When effective, maximum analgesia is obtained within 5 minutes of inhalation. Although the inhalation of nitrous oxide produces a rapid effect on the central nervous system and depresses cortical function, there are no direct effects on the respiratory system. Cough and gag reflexes are not altered. Its extremely short half-life makes it a valuable prehospital medication.

Indications

- Musculoskeletal trauma
- Myocardial infarction
- Thermal burns

Contraindications

- Altered mental status
- Alcohol intoxication
- Head injury
- Abdominal or chest trauma
- Shock
- Pneumothorax
- Pulmonary disease (COPD or asthma)
- Inability to comprehend or respond to verbal commands
- Abdominal distention suggestive of bowel obstruction

Equipment

- Nitronox blender with facemask (Figure 4-28)

Procedure

1. Use universal precautions.

2. Invert the nitrous tank several times to create vaporization.

3. Open the pressure valves on the oxygen and nitrous oxide tanks.

4. Make sure the pressure gauges are reading in the green bands, indicating proper pressure, and record the pressure.

5. Instruct the patient on the use of the device and what effects to anticipate.

6. Place the patient in a sitting position. In-

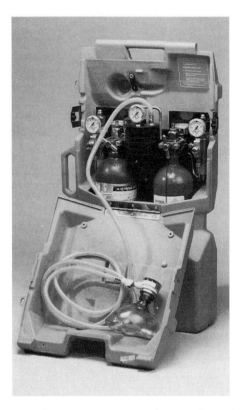

Figure 4-28 Nitronox machine with mask.

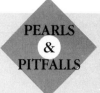

PEARLS & PITFALLS

A Few Precautions...

◆ After sitting for periods of time, nitrous oxide will liquefy in the bottom of the tank. Hence, before using Nitronox, the tank must be inverted several times to re-vaporize the gas.

◆ In the closed space of the ambulance compartment, be aware of ambient nitrous oxide gas that may affect all in the compartment. Patient compartment exhaust fans should be used. When patients receive a high analgesic effect, they frequently will allow the mask to drop from their face.

◆ Monitor vital signs frequently throughout the procedure.

◆ The Nitronox blender has an oxygen fail-safe mechanism that automatically stops the flow of nitrous oxide in the system when the oxygen is depleted.

◆ Nitrous oxide has a high abuse potential. Security systems should be in place.

struct and assist the patient in creating a tight facemask seal.

7. Encourage the patient to inhale and exhale normally. If the patient feels uncomfortable for any reason during the procedure, he or she should simply remove the mask and breathe normally (Figure 4-29).

8. No one should apply the facemask to the patient except the patient himself.

9. Monitor the patient for changes in level of consciousness and other vital signs.

◆ Alternate Intravenous Access Routes—Central Venous Catheters

A central venous catheter (CVC) is any catheter whose proximal tip is positioned in either the inferior vena cava, superior vena cava, or right atrium of the heart.

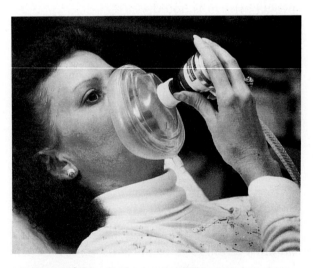

Figure 4-29 Patient using Nitronox, keeping tight facial seal with the mask.

Background

CVCs are not placed by paramedics in the prehospital setting. They are placed under sterile conditions when long-term venous access will be required. Patients with chronic illness who need frequent blood drawings, blood transfusions, hydration therapy, nutritional support, pain management, or chemotherapy are all candidates for CVCs.

Although paramedics do not initiate these catheters, knowledge of them and of how to access each type is essential in today's prehospital setting. Most homebound patients with central catheters have very poor peripheral vasculature. Hence, the prehospital provider can access a CVC with minimal effort, without inflicting undo pain and trauma on the patient. It is suggested that Medical Control/Direction authorize any intervention involving CVCs.

Two basic types of devices are used for long-term home care patients. The Hickman, Broviac, and Groshong catheters are examples of the first type. They are indwelling catheters that are surgically inserted through an incision

in the patient's chest in the deltopectoral groove. The catheter is placed into the superior vena cava, where the proximal tip terminates just above the right atrium of the heart. Most of these catheters are tunneled through the skin, sutured in place, and have the distal end positioned in an area outside of the chest where it is easily accessible to the patient or caregiver (Figure 4-30). Many of these types of indwelling catheters require heparin injections to maintain patency.

The second form of central venous access is implantable catheters. The Mediport, Porta-cath, and Infusaport are examples of this type of catheter (Figure 4-31). The catheter is surgically positioned in the superior vena cava or right atrium by surgical cut down of the cephalic or jugular vein or by percutaneous placement into the subclavian vein. The distal port is then placed under the skin over a bony prominence, such as a rib, clavicle, or sternum. The injection device has a self-sealing silicone rubber port, which allows for multiple sticks. A special subcutaneous needle, known as a Hu-

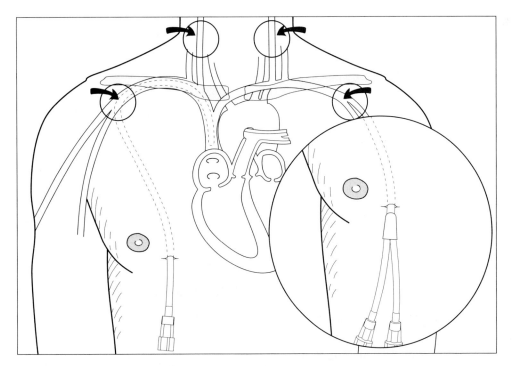

Figure 4-30   Locations for CVC injection ports.

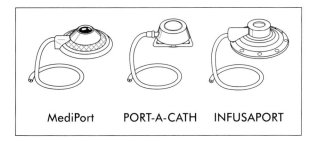

Figure 4-31 Examples of commonly used implanted injection ports.

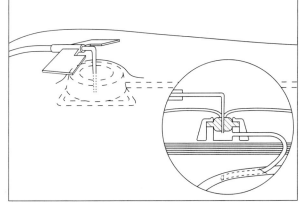

Figure 4-32 Correct placement of a Huber needle into an implantable catheter.

ber needle, must be used to access the device (Figure 4-32). The needles used on most ambulances will not access this style of catheter.

◆ Putting It All Together

One of the most important skills performed by the advanced prehospital provider is medication administration. It is significant to the patient in two ways. First, the rapid administration of a medication can be lifesaving in critical situations. Second, aseptic technique can reduce the length of hospital stay of a patient. Many patients are retained unnecessarily in a hospital as the result of secondary infection. The novice advanced life support provider, as well as the veteran, should periodically go through supervised skills practice and evaluation.

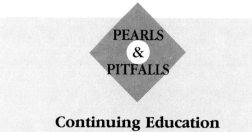

PEARLS & PITFALLS

Continuing Education

It is suggested that you receive education and practice time with each of these devices before accessing them in the field. Again, direct Medical Control/Direction should be contacted when medication and intravenous fluid are given via any route that is not traditionally used in the prehospital setting.

Testing Your Knowledge

1. From the following list, select the the form of injection in which the medication is administered into the "fatty" layer of tissue.

   a. Intradermal
   b. Subcutaneous
   c. Dermal
   d. Intramuscular

2. The most common medication given subcutaneously by prehospital providers is:

   a. Diphenhydramine
   b. Insulin
   c. Epinephrine 1:1,000
   d. Epinephrine 1:10,000

3. Poor perfusion can result in poor absorption of subcutaneously injected medications.

    a. True

    b. False

4. The intramuscular administration of a drug provides a more rapid absorption route when compared with endotracheal or intravenous bolus.

    a. True

    b. False

5. When giving an IM injection, the paramedic should insert the needle into the muscle using which of the following angles of entry?

    a. 15-degree

    b. 45-degree

    c. 70-degree

    d. 90-degree

6. From the following list, select the route that is most commonly used by paramedics for administering drugs in life-threatening situations.

    a. Intravenous bolus (IV push)

    b. Endotracheal bolus

    c. Subcutaneous

    d. Mediport

7. IV piggyback infusion is most suited in the prehospital setting when a medication is required for continuous flow or titration to an effect.

    a. True

    b. False

8. The mnemonic "NAVEL" is used when describing the five medications that can be given via an ETT. List those five drugs.

9. Hyperventilation of the patient should be provided before and after the administration of an endotracheal bolus medication.

    a. True

    b. False

10. Patients receiving nebulized bronchodilators must always be monitored for tachycardia and other dysrhythmias.

    a. True

    b. False

Answers are in Appendix A.

BIBLIOGRAPHY

Caroline NL: *Emergency care in the streets*, ed 3, Boston, 1987, Little, Brown, pp 105, 107-108, 128-130.

Dula DJ: Nitrous oxide analgesia. In Roberts JR, Hedges JR, editors: *Clinical procedures in emergency medicine*, ed 2, Philadelphia, 1991, WB Saunders, pp 508-514.

Field DL, Hedges JR: Noninvasive assessment and delivery of oxygen and inhaled medications. In Roberts JR, Hedges JR, editors: *Clinical procedures in emergency medicine*, ed 2, Philadelphia, 1991, WB Saunders, pp 64-83.

Moldawer NP, Newton M: Administering by the parenteral route. In West RS, editor: *Giving medications*, Horsham, Pa, 1981, Intermed Communications, pp 78-83, 88-94.

New England Critical Care: Patient Education Information, *Your central venous access port.*

New England Critical Care: Patient Education Information, *Your central venous Groshong catheter.*

Stewart RD: Nitrous oxide. In Paris PM, Stewart RD, editors: *Pain Management in emergency medicine*, Norwalk, Conn, 1988, Appleton & Lange, pp 221-238.

Ward JT: Endotracheal drug administration. In Roberts JR, Hedges JR, editors: *Clinical procedures in emergency medicine*, ed 2, Philadelphia, 1991, WB Saunders, pp 369-376.

Subcutaneous (SQ) Injection

Subcutaneous injection is a method of administering a medication directly into the subcutaneous tissue, where it is absorbed into the general circulation.

Procedure	Possible points	Points awarded
Observe universal precautions.	1	
Confirm drug order, route, and amount.	3	
Explain procedure and reconfirm that patient is not allergic to drug.	2	
Check drug name, expiration, and coloration.	3	
Assemble equipment.	1	
Calculate and draw up desired volume of medication into syringe.	2	
Eject any air from syringe.	1	
Identify appropriate injection site.	1	
Cleanse site with alcohol or povidone-iodine.	1	
"Tent" skin and advise patient to prepare for a stick.	2	
Insert needle at 45-degree angle into subcutaneous tissue.	1	
Aspirate syringe, checking for air or blood.	1	
Slowly inject medication.	1	
Withdraw needle and apply pressure to site with sterile gauze pad.	2	
Properly dispose of syringe and medication container.	1	
Monitor patient for drug effect.	1	
TOTAL POINTS	**24**	

COMMENTS _____

Intramuscular (IM) Injection

Intramuscular injection is a method of administering a medication directly into the muscle, where it is subsequently absorbed into the general circulation.

Procedure	Possible points	Points awarded
Observe universal precautions.	1	
Confirm drug order, amount, and route.	3	
Explain procedure and reconfirm that patient is not allergic to drug.	2	
Check drug name, expiration, and coloration.	3	
Assemble equipment.	1	
Calculate and draw up desired volume of medication into syringe.	2	
Eject any air from syringe.	1	
Identify appropriate injection site.	1	
Cleanse site with alcohol or povidone-iodine.	1	
Stretch or "flatten" skin overlying site with your fingers and tell patient to prepare for a stick.	2	
Insert needle at 90-degree angle into muscle.	1	
Aspirate syringe, checking for air or blood.	1	
Slowly inject medication.	1	
Withdraw needle and apply pressure to site with sterile gauze pad.	2	
Properly dispose of syringe and medication container.	1	
Monitor patient for drug effect.	1	
TOTAL POINTS	**24**	

COMMENTS _____

_____

_____

Intravenous Bolus (IV Push)

Intravenous bolus, or "IV push," is a method of administering a drug directly into the vein, allowing for a rapid onset of medication.

Procedure (assumes IV has been established)	Possible points	Points awarded
Observe universal precautions.	1	
Confirm drug order, amount, and route.	3	
Explain procedure and reconfirm that patient is not allergic to drug.	2	
Check drug name, expiration, and coloration.	3	
Assemble equipment.	1	
Calculate and draw up desired volume of medication into syringe.	2	
Eject any air from syringe.	1	
Cleanse rubber injection port on IV tubing with alcohol.	1	
Insert needle into rubber injection port.	1	
Pinch off IV tubing just above injection port.	1	
Inject desired amount of medication according to recommendations into injection port.	1	
Release (unpinch) IV tubing.	1	
Flush IV tubing with fluid.	1	
Readjust IV flow rate.	1	
Properly dispose of syringe and medication container.	1	
Monitor patient for medication effect.	1	
TOTAL POINTS	22	

COMMENTS

Intravenous Drip Infusion (Intravenous Piggyback)

IV piggyback (IVPB) provides a route for continuous administration of a medication. This is accomplished by connecting an intravenous infusion containing a medication to a preexisting IV site.

Procedure (assumes IV has been established)	Possible points	Points awarded
Observe universal precautions.	1	
Confirm drug order, amount, and route.	3	
Explain procedure and reconfirm that patient is not allergic to drug.	2	
Check drug name, expiration, and coloration.	3	
Calculate and draw up desired volume of drug into syringe.	2	
Check IV fluid for clarity and proper fluid.	1	
Cleanse injection port on IV bag or bottle with alcohol prep.	1	
Insert needle into injection port on bag or bottle, and inject medication.	1	
Mix drug in IV solution by gently shaking bag or bottle.	1	
Place medication label on bag or bottle.	1	
Attach administration set and purge IV tubing of air.	1	
Attach needle to end of administration set, clean nearest injection port to patient, and attach IVPB.	3	
Properly dispose of syringe and medication container.	1	
Calculate and adjust flow rate for both primary and secondary IV.	2	
Secure patient for medication effect.	1	
TOTAL POINTS	**24**	

COMMENTS _____

_____

_____

Endotracheal Bolus

Endotracheal bolus is a procedure that allows the delivery of a medication directly to the tracheobronchial tree and lung tissue, via an ETT.

Procedure	Possible points	Points awarded
Observe universal precautions.	1	
Confirm drug order, amount, and route.	3	
Check drug name, expiration, and coloration.	3	
Assemble syringe (medications for endotracheal route are almost always provided in prefilled syringes).	1	
Calculate desired volume of medication.	1	
Hyperventilate patient.	1	
Disconnect bag-valve device from ETT (stop chest compressions).	1	
Insert needle into lumen of ETT and forcefully inject medication.	1	
Reconnect bag-valve device and hyperventilate patient for 10 seconds.	1	
Resume appropriate ventilation and chest compressions.	1	
Reverify ETT placement.	1	
Monitor patient for medication effect.	1	
TOTAL POINTS	16	

COMMENTS _____

_____

_____

Nebulized Inhalation

Nebulized inhalation of medication is a method of delivering a drug via the tracheobronchial tree, using a device known as a nebulizer.

Procedure	Possible points	Points awarded
Observe universal precautions.	1	
Explain procedure to patient.	1	
Establish baseline vital signs and connect patient to cardiac monitor.	2	
Assemble equipment. Place bronchodilator and saline solution in reservoir well of nebulizer.	2	
Connect nebulizer to oxygen source and adjust oxygen flow.	1	
Encourage patient to inhale normally, having patient take a deep breath every 3 to 5 inhalations.	1	
Discontinue treatment when solution is depleted.	1	
Place patient on supplemental oxygen following medication administration.	1	
Monitor vital signs and patient for medication effect.	2	
TOTAL POINTS	**12**	

COMMENTS _____

_____

_____

Self-Administered Nitrous Oxide (Nitronox)

Nitronox is a 50:50 mixture of nitrous oxide and oxygen, which is self-administered by the patient.

Procedure	Possible points	Points awarded
Observe universal precautions.	1	
Invert nitrous tank several times to create vaporization.	1	
Open pressure valves on oxygen and nitrous tanks.	1-	
Record pressure in tanks.	1	
Instruct patient on use of device and what effects to anticipate.	2	
Assist patient in creating and maintaining tight facial mask seal.	1	
Encourage patient to inhale and exhale normally.	1	
Monitor patient for changes in level of consciousness and other vital signs.	1	
TOTAL POINTS	9	

COMMENTS _____

_____

_____

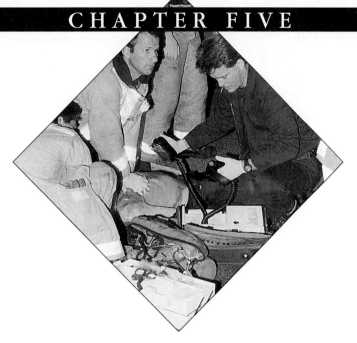

CHAPTER FIVE

Cardiac Skills

Objectives

A paramedic should be able to—

1. Discuss the electrical conduction of the heart and the significance of each wave.

2. Identify parts of the EKG monitor/ defibrillator and the significance of each part.

3. Be able to properly apply EKG leads.

4. List and demonstrate the procedure for using quick-look paddles.

5. List and demonstrate the steps necessary for proper EKG lead application and cardiac monitoring of a patient.

6. Define and differentiate between defibrillation and synchronized cardioversion.

7. List two safety concerns when defibrillating or cardioverting a patient.

8. Identify two rhythms that would require defibrillation.

9. Demonstrate on a mannequin the steps necessary for proper defibrillation.

10. List two indications for use of synchronized cardioversion.

11. Demonstrate on a mannequin the proper technique for synchronized cardioversion.

12. Define and give examples of three types of vagal maneuvers.

13. List three indications and contraindications for vagal maneuvers.

14. Demonstrate on a mannequin the proper procedure for patient assessment and performance of various vagal maneuvers.

15. Define noninvasive pacing.

16. List two indications for the use of noninvasive pacing.

17. Demonstrate on a mannequin the proper technique for noninvasive pacing.

Case Scenario

You are called one evening to a local adult care facility for a patient who has fallen. You arrive to find a 77-year-old male lying on the floor with a pillow placed under his head. He was walking down the hallway when he "simply passed out." He complains of weakness and dizziness, especially when he stands, and has a small hematoma on his right forearm. His weakness appears to have been occurring periodically for 2 days. This gentleman has experienced some anginal pain and two episodes of congestive heart failure within the last 5 years. He routinely takes Lanoxin and Nitrostat. Vital signs note that the patient is alert and oriented; heart rate is 40, weak and regular; respiratory rate is 28 and shallow; blood pressure is 78/56; EKG shows third-degree heart block; and pulse oximetry notes saturation at 93%. There are no additional signs of acute illness or injury.

You establish high-flow oxygen via nonrebreathing mask soon after you arrive. You initiate an intravenous line (IV) of D_5W in the patient's left forearm, using an 18-gauge catheter, and infuse it at a keep-open rate. Since the patient appears to be experiencing symptomatic bradycardia secondary to third-degree heart block, medical direction is sought. Atropine 0.5 mg is requested and granted. A repeat bolus is suggested if no improvement is noted. Furthermore, external cardiac pacing is granted if the atropine fails.

Following the second bolus of atropine, the patient's rate is still unchanged. You connect the patient to the noninvasive pacer by applying one large patch to the anterior chest over the left ventricle and one patch to the posterior chest between the scapulae. The rate is set at 80 beats per minute, and the milliamperes set at 70. You turn the pacer on and note some muscle twitching on the patient's chest; however, his heart rate does not improve. After 1 minute, the milliamperes are increased to 80. The patient states that he is experiencing some discomfort but feels better. His pulse is at 80, and capture has been obtained. BP is 114/78. Medical direction recommends diazepam 3 mg IV slow push to help the patient relax and produce mild amnesia.

Transport to the medical center occurs without any complications. The patient is presented to the emergency department in good condition, where a temporary transvenous pacer is inserted. The following day, he receives a permanent pacemaker and returns to the adult care facility after a short hospital stay.

Cardiac care has become an important aspect of prehospital emergency medicine. With the advancement of technology and pharmacology, a paramedic has the skill and tools to treat many conditions that 10 years ago if left untreated could have resulted in the patient's death. However, it must be remembered that an EKG monitor is just another tool that assists us in evaluating our patients. **It must never replace a paramedic's assessment of cardiac function.**

The skills covered in this chapter deal with those that you may use in various cardiac emergencies. The use of the EKG monitor/defibrillator, including lead application and quick-look monitoring; synchronized cardioversion; noninvasive cardiac pacing; and vagal maneuvers, is discussed. Medical direction may be required by some EMS systems before initiating these procedures.

◆ The EKG Monitor/ Defibrillator/Pacer and Cardiac Monitoring

The electrocardiogram (ECG or EKG) is the reproduction of the electrical activity of the heart on graph paper to allow for interpretation of cardiac rhythm.

Background

The basic piece of equipment in cardiac care is the monitor/ defibrillator. Recently, with the advent of prehospital noninvasive (external) cardiac pacing, these devices have taken on a new look. Many units have now been modified to include the pacer component.

Cardiac Monitors

Component	Function
Cardioscope	Displays EKG
	Trace moves left to right
Defibrillator	Delivers electrical current to the heart
Recorder	Records EKG onto paper
	Recording is delayed by approximately 2.4 seconds
Freeze (push)	Momentary pushbutton that freezes the cardioscope tracing (Figure 5-1)
EKG size	Button that controls the height of the EKG complex on both the scope and recorder
Record (push)	Pushbutton switch that provides power to the recorder (Figure 5-2)
CAL (push)	Momentary pushbutton switch that gives 1 mV calibrating pulse to monitor, recorder, and EKG output (Figure 5-3)
QRS vol	Button that controls the volume of the systolic beeper (Figure 5-4)

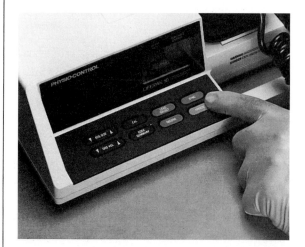

Figure 5-1   Freeze button.

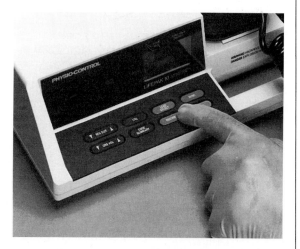

Figure 5-2   Record button.

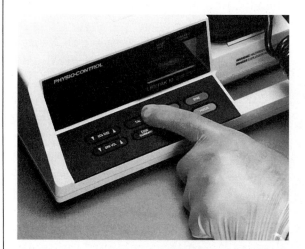

Figure 5-3   Calibration "CAL" button.

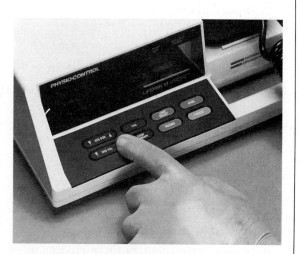

Figure 5-4   QRS volume button.

Continued.

Cardiac Monitors—cont'd

Component	Function
Power	Switch for main power to the monitor
Three-lead pa-tient cable	Where monitoring cable connects
Lead select button	Allows the operator to select between three leads (lead I, II, or III) for viewing the electrical activity of the heart from different angles (Figure 5-5)
EKG out	1 volt EKG output jack that is used for modular or radio/modulator
Low battery indicator light	Flashing red light indicates a low battery **CHANGE BATTERY WHEN FLASHING**
Battery pak	Nicad battery pak
Noninvasive external cardiac pacemaker (optional)	Device that allows for the external application of low-ampere electrical stimulation in bradycardic heart rhythms

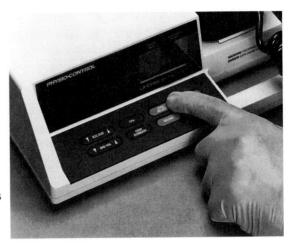

Figure 5-5   Lead selection button.

Indications

♦ EKG monitoring is indicated for any critical patient, any patient who gives a cardiac or respiratory history, or any patient who gives a medical history that does not correlate with symptomatology.

Contraindications

♦ None

Lead placement and cardiac monitoring

Field monitoring of the EKG differs from in-hospital 12-lead EKG tracing. EKG monitoring in the field uses only three electrodes. Generally, leads I, II, III are used. Some systems use the modified chest lead I (MCL I) position. The monitoring device requires three electrodes: a positive, a negative, and a ground. Each moni-toring view is simply a variation of electrode placement.

Lead II usually provides the best picture of the electrical activity of the heart because its position is quite similar to the normal electrical axis of the heart (Figure 5-6). MCL I is particularly useful when monitoring for the presence of ectopic beats.

When placing electrodes on the chest for monitoring purposes, place them high enough on the shoulders and low enough on the chest to avoid the apex of the heart. The white and black electrodes should be positioned just below the clavicle bilaterally, and the red electrode is placed at the lower edge of the left rib cage near the anterior axillary line. If the patient has a permanent implanted cardiac pacemaker, be sure to avoid placing EKG electrodes

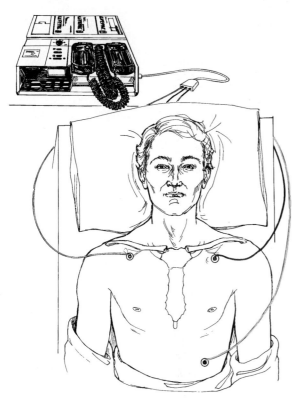

Figure 5-6 Lead placement.

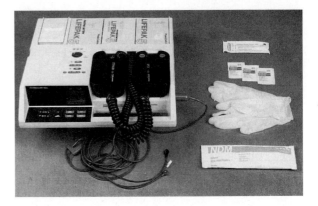

Figure 5-7 Equipment for monitoring.

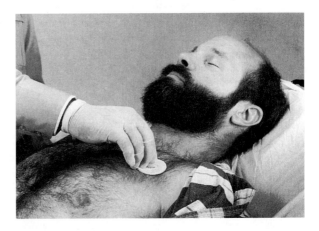

Figure 5-8 Place the leads.

over the battery pack so that, should it become necessary to defibrillate the patient, there will be room on the chest wall for the two defibrillator paddles (sternum and apex) without moving electrodes.

Equipment (Figure 5-7)

- EKG monitor
- Disposable electrodes
- EKG lead cables

Procedure

1. Explain to your patient what you are going to do and why.

2. Peel off the paper backing on the electrode. Check to make sure the center of the electrode is moist with conductive jelly. If the sponge is dry, discard the electrode because a poor EKG signal will result.

3. Place the electrode at the chosen site with the adhesive side down. Apply pressure at the center of the electrode, moving outward, to ensure a good seal (Figure 5-8).

4. Attach the monitor cables to electrodes. The electrodes will either be marked with RA, RL, LA abbreviation; or +, -, G symbols; or they will be color coded. You must know your system's markings (Figure 5-9).

5. Connect the leads to the EKG monitor.

6. Turn the monitor on and select the proper lead (Figure 5-10).

7. Observe the monitor (Figure 5-11) and adjust the EKG size to the desired height. The QRS should be high enough to visualize and create a "beep" sound when the volume is increased (Figure 5-12).

8. Adjust systolic volume to desired volume (Figure 5-13).

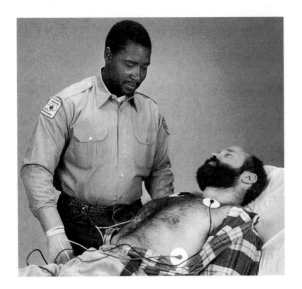

Figure 5-9 Correct lead placement.

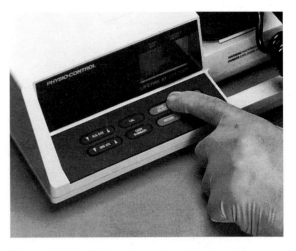

Figure 5-10 Select the proper lead.

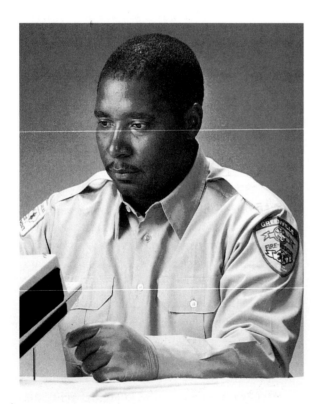

Figure 5-11 Observe the monitor.

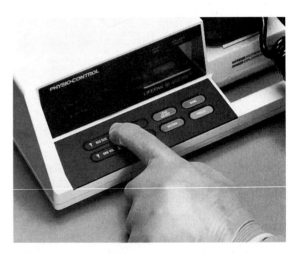

Figure 5-12 Adjust the size of the EKG.

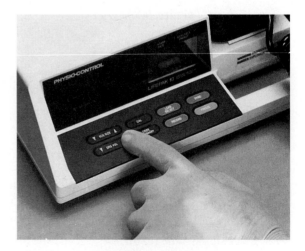

Figure 5-13 Adjust the volume.

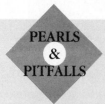

PEARLS & PITFALLS

"The Electrodes Won't Stick!"

Unfortunately, EKG electrodes do not always stick to the patient or stay where they are placed. Similarly, in critical patients, you may not have time to be chasing loose electrodes around the back of the ambulance. Listed below are three methods that may help you to keep electrodes where they belong:

• Clean the patient's skin with an alcohol prep to remove the body's natural oils and dirt. Once the skin is dry, lightly abrade the skin with a 4 × 4.

• Apply a light coat of benzoin to the skin and allow it to dry for approximately 30 seconds. Benzoin becomes very sticky when drying.

• Spray a light layer of your favorite powdered antiperspirant to the skin and allow it to dry for 30 seconds. Then wipe the powder away. The remaining antiperspirant will absorb moisture for the short duration and allow the electrode to stick with ease.

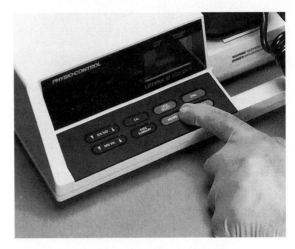

Figure 5-14 Record a 6-second strip for the patient's chart.

9. Press the record button and run a tracing of the patient's rhythm. A minimum of 6 seconds is needed for each copy of the patient's chart (Figure 5-14).

10. Label the EKG strip with the patient's name, date and time.

Use of Quick-Look Paddles

When the paramedic arrives at a scene and finds a pulseless, nonbreathing patient, he or she may use quick-look paddles to ascertain the patient's cardiac rhythm. By using the quick-look paddles, the patient can be rapidly defibrillated if ventricular fibrillation or pulseless ventricular tachycardia is found.

Procedure

1. Turn on the EKG monitor.

2. Turn the lead selector to PADDLES.

3. Apply conductive gel to paddles or use specifically designed defibrillation gel pads (Figure 5-15, *A* and *B*)

4. Place paddles firmly on the bare chest with the paddle marked STERNUM on the patient's right chest near the sternum and the paddle marked APEX on the patient's lower left chest (Figure 5-16).

5. Adjust EKG size to the desired height (Figure 5-17).

6. Observe the scope and determine the patient's condition (Figure 5-18). Check pulse and verify absence of pulse.

7. If potentially fatal ventricular dysrhythmia is noted, proceed with the defibrillation algorithm.

8. Remember, this method is for a quick-look and initial defibrillation only. It is not meant to be used for continuous patient monitoring; hence, following the initial three defibrillation attempts, the patient should be connected to the EKG monitor using traditional leads.

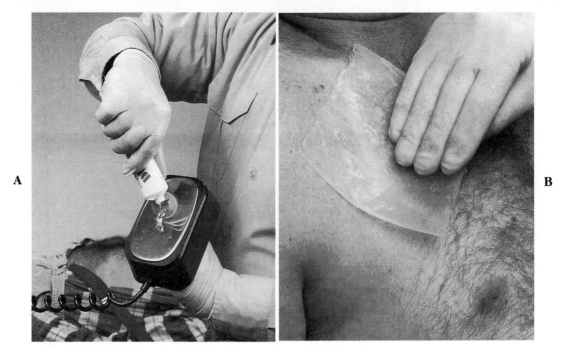

Figure 5-15 **A**, Apply conductive gel. **B**, Apply defibrillation pads.

Table 5-1 Troubleshooting Your EKG Monitor

Trouble	Probable cause
Unit does not function when power applied	Battery low or dead
Interference on cardioscope when using patient cable	Poor electrode contact
	Defective patient cable
	Poor skin preparation
	Dried electrode gel
	Power/mode selection in PADDLES
Excessive interference when using quick-look paddles	Defective or dirty paddles
	Poor paddle contact with skin
	Inadequate conductive gel
	Cable motion
No EKG signal on cardioscope when using patient cables, but calibration on display is available	Defective patient cables
	Power/mode selection in PADDLES
	Cables not inserted tightly
No EKG signal on cardioscope when using paddles, but calibration on display is available	Defective paddles
	Power/mode selection in EKG LEAD
	Defibrillator and monitor not attached securely to each other (Lifepak 5)
	Power/mode selection on LEAD I, II, or III
Recorder does not run	Battery low
	Defective paper drive motor
Recorder motor runs but does not print rhythm strip	Stylus heat too low
	Stylus bent or maladjusted
Monitor shows a straight line only	EKG size is turned down
	Power/mode selection in PADDLES

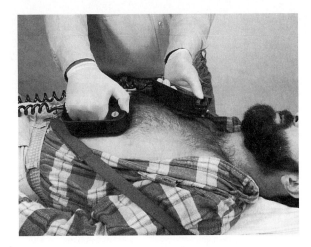

Figure 5-16 Correct paddle placement.

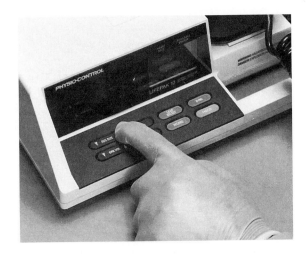

Figure 5-17 Adjust the EKG size.

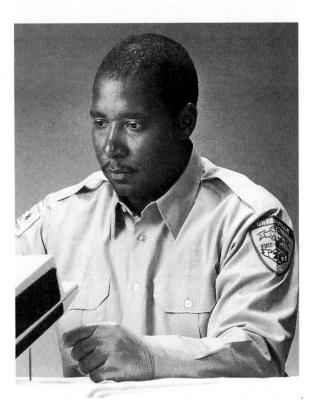

Figure 5-18 Observe the monitor.

◆ Defibrillation

Defibrillation, also known as unsynchronized countershock, is the random delivery of high-intensity electrical charge to a fibrillating heart. The purpose of this charge is to depolarize the myocardium and restore the sinoatrial (SA) node as the dominant pacemaker.

Background

Ventricular fibrillation and pulseless ventricular tachycardia are potentially fatal dysrhythmias characterized by electrical and mechanical chaos. These dysrhythmias may occur in the presence of coronary artery disease, electrical shock, drowning, drug overdose, or acid/base disturbance. There is only one definitive treatment for ventricular fibrillation and pulseless ventricular tachycardia: defibrillation.

Most defibrillators are very simple to use. It is essential to become familiar with the defibrillator that is used in your department, since it may work a little differently from the one shown in this textbook.

Equipment (Figure 5-19)
* Monitor/defibrillator
* Monitor leads
* Defibrillator pads or conductive gel

Procedure
1. Establish unresponsiveness.
2. Check to make sure patient is pulseless and not breathing (Figure 5-20).

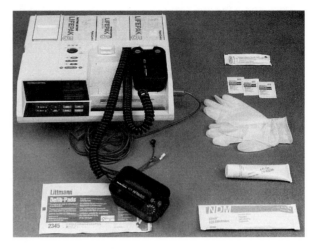

Figure 5-19 Equipment needed for defibrillation.

PEARLS & PITFALLS

Successful Defibrillation

A paramedic can make defibrillation attempts more successful if the following points are remembered:

• Speed is of utmost importance if defibrillation is to be successful. The longer the time period between the onset of fibrillation and defibrillation, the less the likelihood of success.

• Paddle placement must be placed so that the ventricles are in the current path. Electricity is known to follow the path of least resistance. This path corresponds to the coronary circulation and the electrical system of the heart.

• Bone is a poor conductor; therefore, paddles should not be placed directly over the sternum.

• Resistance to current flow will decrease with each successive defibrillation, especially if the time interval between each shock is short.

• Always maintain an adequate airway to correct hypoxia and acidosis. Heart muscle that is deprived of oxygen is difficult to defibrillate into a viable and perfusing rhythm.

• Never shock a patient on a wet surface! The current may follow the residual water, resulting in an uneffective delivery of current, burns to the patient, or defibrillation of the medic or bystanders.

• Do not shock over nitroglycerin paste or a pacemaker battery pack.

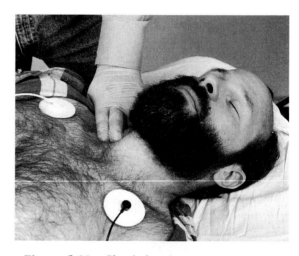

Figure 5-20 Check for absence of pulse and breathlessness.

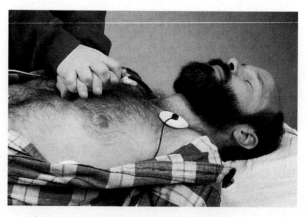

Figure 5-21 Begin CPR if the patient has no pulse.

3. Have someone begin CPR while you prepare the defibrillator (Figure 5-21).

4. Turn the monitor/defibrillator to the ON position (first battery) and select the PADDLE mode in preparation for using quick-look paddles (Figure 5-22).

5. Note that "0" appears under AVAILABLE ENERGY.

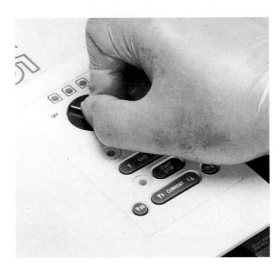

Figure 5-22 Turn the power selector to the ON position.

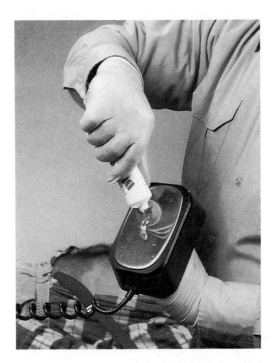

Figure 5-23 Apply defibrillation gel or pads.

6. Apply the conductive medium (Figure 5-23). Defibrillation gel or pads may be used. The conductive material conducts electricity and at the same time reduces the risk of electrical burns. DO NOT use alcohol-soaked pads because they may ignite! If using conductive gel on the paddles, make sure the entire surface of the paddle is covered with jelly by rubbing them together (Figure 5-24). Take care not to rub paddles so hard that jelly oozes onto sides of the paddles or your hands. If that happens, remove excess jelly with a cloth before proceeding.

7. Select the correct electrical charge on defibrillator paddles. (Figure 5-25).

8. Press the charge button and release.

9. Place the paddles firmly on the chest, exerting 20 to 25 pounds of pressure. Place one paddle on the right of the sternum between the second and third intercostal space and the other at the fifth intercostal space, left midclavicular line, near the apex of the heart (Figure 5-26).

10. The defibrillator is ready to fire when the charge indicator light stops flashing and glows steadily. The defibrillator will not fire unless it is fully charged to the desired energy level.

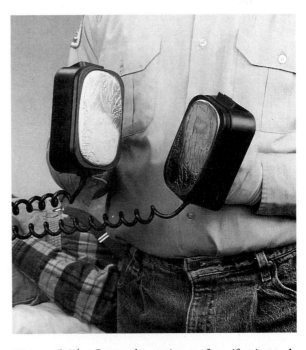

Figure 5-24 Cover the entire surface if using gel.

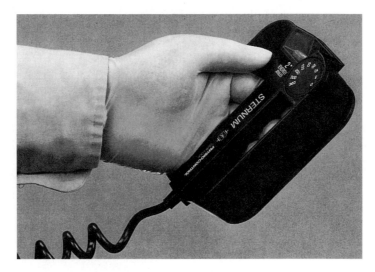

Figure 5-25   Select the proper joule setting.

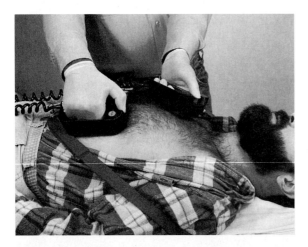

Figure 5-26   Place paddles on the chest.

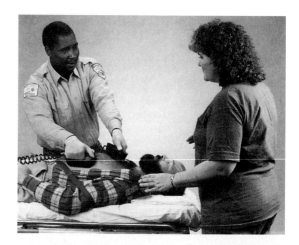

Figure 5-27   Call "CLEAR" and visualize the area.

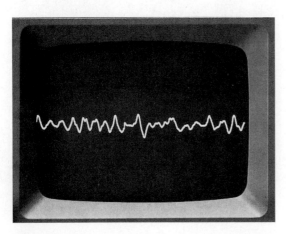

Figure 5-28   Confirm ventricular fibrillation.

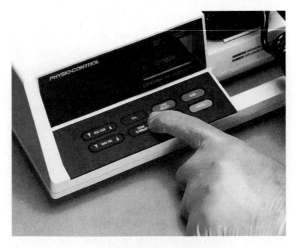

Figure 5-29   Document the events of the arrest by pushing the CODE SUMMARY button.

11. Call "CLEAR" and visually clear the area to verify that no one, including yourself, is in contact with the patient (Figure 5-27).

12. Check monitor screen one more time before defibrillating to make sure the patient is still in ventricular fibrillation (Figure 5-28).

13. Depress **both** paddle discharge buttons **simultaneously** for defibrillation.

14. Check the patient's EKG strip to see if ventricular fibrillation was terminated and have a co-worker check a pulse.

15. If repeat defibrillation is indicated, depress CHARGE and repeat the above steps according to the algorithms.

16. Document the procedure. Documentation should include:

    a. EKG strip of defibrillation - push CODE SUMMARY on the Life-Pak 10 (Figure 5-29).

    b. Patient's name, date, time, lead, joules delivered, and number of defibrillations (Figure 5-30).

    c. Postdefibrillation rhythm

17. If further defibrillation is unnecessary, be sure that there is no charge in the defibrillator. Most defibrillators "dump" their charge into the machine by turning the joules selection dial to another setting.

18. Once the machine is disarmed, quickly clean the paddles by wiping them with a paper towel or 4 × 4 gauze pad. Once at the hospital, the paddles must be cleaned with soap and water. Make sure all conductive jelly is removed because any jelly that remains may corrode and pit the paddle heads, which may cause electrical arcing and skin burns in the future (Figure 5-31).

19. Contact and advise Medical Control of the patient's status (Figure 5-32).

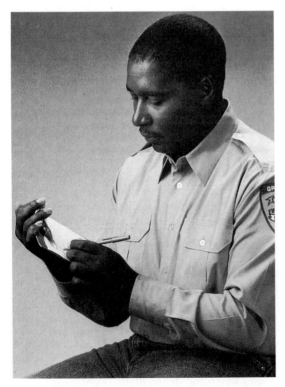

Figure 5-30 Document the patient's name, date, lead, joules delivered, number of shocks, and post-defibrillation rhythm.

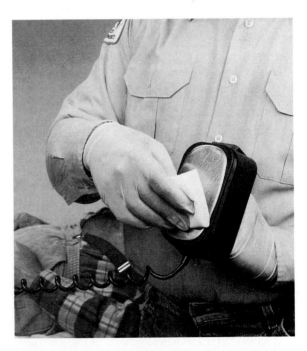

Figure 5-31 Clean paddles if gel was used.

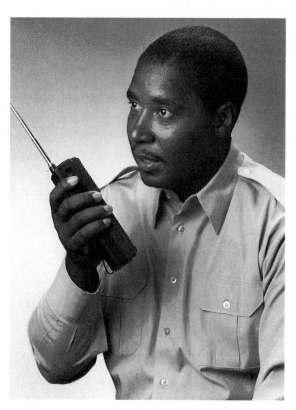

Figure 5-32 Advise Medical Control of the patient's status.

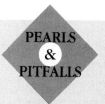

PEARLS
&
PITFALLS

Pediatric Electrical Therapy

Ventricular fibrillation is uncommon in children and rare in infants. Cardiac arrest in the pediatric population is most often secondary to respiratory arrest. However, if defibrillation is necessary on a child, begin at 2 J/kg and repeat at 4 J/kg. Cardioversion is performed at 1 J/kg, and repeated at 2 J/kg.

Pediatric paddles should be used whenever possible when performing electrical therapy. If unavailable, adult paddles can be used by placing the child on his or her side and using an anterior-posterior approach.

Table 5-2 Troubleshooting Your Defibrillator

Trouble	Probable cause/solution
The defibrillator may not discharge if:	
Wrong buttons are pressed.	Some defibrillators have an on/off button on one paddle and a charge button on the other paddle. These buttons are sometimes used inadvertently instead of the proper discharge button. When the wrong button is pushed, the charge is dumped, causing a delay in defibrillation.
Battery is low or dead.	Always make sure to follow the manufacturer's instructions regarding battery maintenance. Carry two fully charged spares in your jump bag. Check the defibrillator each shift to ensure that it is functional. Remember that nicad batteries must be exercised routinely.
Synchronizer button is activated.	If the SYNC button is activated, the monitor will search for QRS complexes. Since the monitor will not be able to locate a QRS complex in V-fib, the defibrillator will not be able to fire.
ENERGY JOULES selector position is changed.	If the joule select is changed while the defibrillator is charging (or after it has charged), the charge is automatically dumped. It then becomes necessary to recharge the unit.

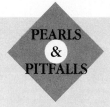

Nicad Batteries

Many prehospital devices such as portable radios, pagers, and cardiac monitor/defibrillators operate on nicad batteries. To "keep them healthy," they must be exercised. Most cardiac monitor/defibrillator batteries should be exercised every 90 days. It is recommended that you read your operator's manual to find out exactly what the manufacturer suggests.

Monitor/defibrillator maintenance

Many details of defibrillator maintenance are specific to the brand that is purchased; instructions should be received from the service representative. Some general defibrillator features should be checked daily:

- Check the roll of paper in the monitor's chart recorder.
- Replace electrodes and defibrillation pads from a fresh, unopened package.
- Make sure that any gel is removed from the paddles, especially the stainless steel paddle surface. Dried gel may pit the paddles and result in uneven distribution and arcing of the current.
- Care for batteries according to the manufacturer's instructions. Replace low batteries before next run.
- Check calibration and energy output according to the manufacturer's instructions.
- Check the defibrillator at least every 24 hours and document.

◆ Synchronized Cardioversion

Cardioversion is the delivery of an electrical shock, timed to the heart's electrical activity, to avoid the relative refractory period. It is designed to interrupt an ectopic pacemaker so that the sinus node can regain control. The monitor/defibrillator senses the R-wave of the EKG and discharges at that point.

Indications

- Supraventricular and ventricular tachydysrhythmias that result in decompensation of the patient (e.g., perfusing ventricular tachycardia, rapid atrial fibrillation, 2:1 atrial flutter)

Contraindications

- Idiojunctional or idioventricular rhythms, as well as second- and third-degree block
- Patients taking certain cardiac drugs (such as digitalis), since these make the patient more disposed to serious complications such as asystole

Equipment (Figure 5-33)

- BP cuff
- Stethoscope
- EKG monitor and leads
- Conductive material
- Bag-valve resuscitator
- Sedative (optional)
- Gloves

Procedure

1. Confirm the presence of the dysrhythmia and the patient's hemodynamic status.
2. Explain the procedure to the patient (Figure 5-34).
3. Establish an IV line, if not already established.
4. Run an EKG strip to document patient's rhythm: label the patient's name, date, and time.
5. Premedicate with sedation as ordered. Be prepared to assist ventilation if necessary.
6. Turn on the defibrillator.
7. Set the defibrillator in the cardiovert mode by depressing the SYNC button. This may vary slightly on different models, so famil-

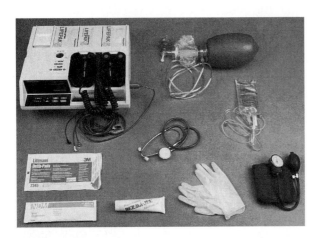

Figure 5-33 Equipment used for synchronized cardioversion.

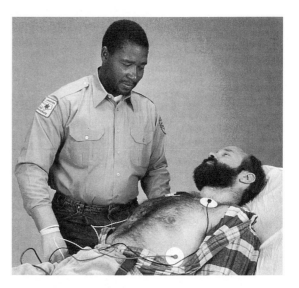

Figure 5-34 Explain the procedure to the patient.

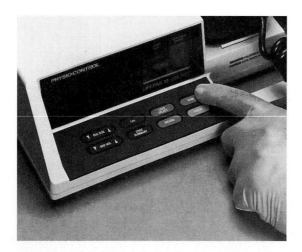

Figure 5-35 Depress the SYNC button.

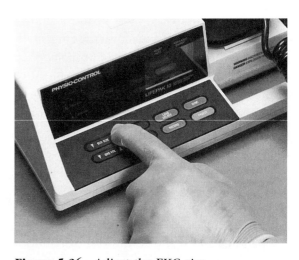

Figure 5-36 Adjust the EKG size.

iarize yourself with your machine. Initial energy delivered should be 50 J (Figure 5-35).

8. Examine the EKG rhythm strip again, making sure that the R-wave is at least 3 cm high. If it isn't, adjust the EKG size (gain) button until it is. The R-wave must be tall enough to trigger the cardioverter (Figure 5-36).

9. Set the control panel to the correct number of joules or watt-seconds.

10. Place defibrillation pads on the patient's

chest or apply conductive gel to paddles (Figure 5-37).

11. Push the charge button. Ensure that the synchronizer is still on and is "marking" the R-wave. Marking the R-waves is recognized by a small light on each R-wave on the cardioscope.

12. Turn the recorder on to record the present rhythm and the effect of the cardioversion (Figure 5-38).

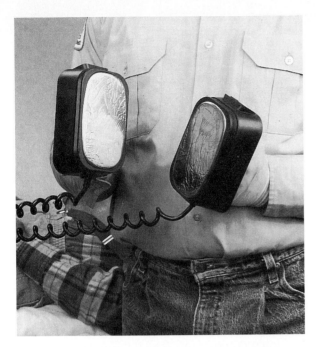

Figure 5-37 Apply defibrillation gel or pads.

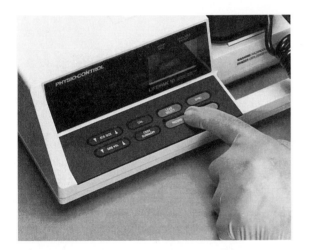

Figure 5-38 Start the rhythm recorder.

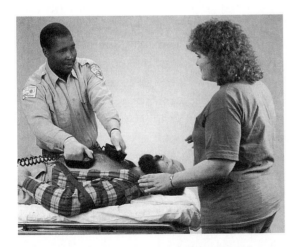

Figure 5-39 Call "CLEAR" and visualize the area.

13. Position the paddles on the chest as you would for defibrillation: one paddle on the right side of the sternum below the clavicle and the other on the left side of the chest at the fifth intercostal space, midclavicular line.

14. Call CLEAR and visualize the area to verify that no one, including yourself, is in contact with the patient (Figure 5-39).

15. Simultaneously press and hold both discharge buttons until the countershock is delivered. There may be a momentary delay while the machine detects the next R-wave.

16. Check the patient's vital signs and level of consciousness. If the patient deteriorates into ventricular fibrillation or pulseless ventricular tachycardia, prepare for immediate defibrillation.

17. Document the entire procedure and rhythm strip (Figure 5-40).

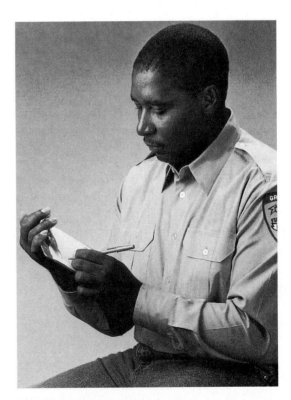

Figure 5-40 Document the patient's name, date, lead, joules delivered, number of shocks, and post-cardioversion rhythm.

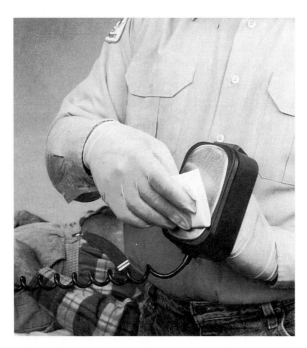

Figure 5-41 Clean paddles if gel was used.

18. If repeat cardioversion is required, repeat steps 7 through 17. If it is not necessary to repeat the procedure, turn off the power. Clean paddles with soap and water to prevent corrosion (Figure 5-41).

◆ Vagal Maneuvers

Vagal maneuvers stimulate the vagus nerve (cranial nerve X), causing a slowing of the sinus node and a decrease in conduction through the AV junction. Vagal stimulation can be used in supraventricular tachycardias as an effective method of slowing or even converting these dysrhythmias to a more stable rhythm.

Background

Two forms of vagal maneuver are used most commonly in the field: Valsalva's maneuver and carotid sinus massage. Both of these methods can be potentially lethal and should be performed with medical direction.

Valsalva's Maneuver

The vagus nerve is stimulated by having the patient hold his or her breath and bear down as if having a bowel movement. This is the most convenient maneuver. Although this appears to be a simple procedure, severe bradydysrhythmias or asystole may occur. The patient and the EKG must be monitored closely before, during, and after the procedure. The patient should be oxygenated and an IV line should be established before the procedure. Have the patient stop immediately if the rhythm slows. Be prepared to resuscitate the patient if necessary. If the Valsalva maneuver fails to convert the patient, be prepared to proceed to carotid sinus massage as directed by Medical Control.

Carotid Sinus Massage

Carotid sinus massage is a noninvasive method of stimulating the vagus nerve and is often effective in slowing tachydysrhythmias.

The vagus nerve is the tenth cranial nerve and is responsible for carrying parasympathetic nerve fibers to the heart and other organs. As the vagus nerve exits the brain, it passes through the neck in close proximity to the carotid artery. You can stimulate the vagus nerve manually by applying firm, steady pressure on the carotid artery near the angle of the jaw, causing the heart rate to decrease.

Indications

Vagal maneuvers are indicated in the treatment of symptomatic supraventricular tachycardia.

Contraindications

Carotid sinus massage should not be performed on patients who are >65 years of age, who have known carotid artery disease, or who have a history of a cerebrovascular accident. It should be standard practice to always palpate both carotid arteries separately to check for equal pulses and to auscultate for bruits in elderly individuals before performing carotid sinus massage.

Complications

Bradydysrhythmias or asystole may occur following vagal maneuvers caused by increased vagal tone. A disruption of carotid plaque may result in a cerebral embolus, causing a cerebrovascular accident.

Equipment (Figure 5-42)

* EKG monitor
* IV D_5W, KVO
* Oxygen
* ACLS equipment

Procedure

1. After evaluating the patient, receive orders from Medical Control.

2. Place the patient on oxygen. Ensure that an IV is established and that the patient is placed on the EKG monitor.

3. Prepare all ACLS equipment.

4. Place the patient in a supine position with head hyperextended. Check the equality of the carotid pulses by gently palpating both arteries **separately**. If the pulse is absent or weak on one side, do not perform the procedure and report to Medical Control (Figure 5-43).

5. Auscultate for bruits, or vascular turbulence, by listening with the bell of the stethoscope over each carotid artery. If bruits are present, do not proceed (Figure 5-44).

6. On the right side of the neck, locate the carotid artery, which is found in a straight line laterally from the larynx (Figure 5-45).

7. Turn the patient's head slightly to the left.

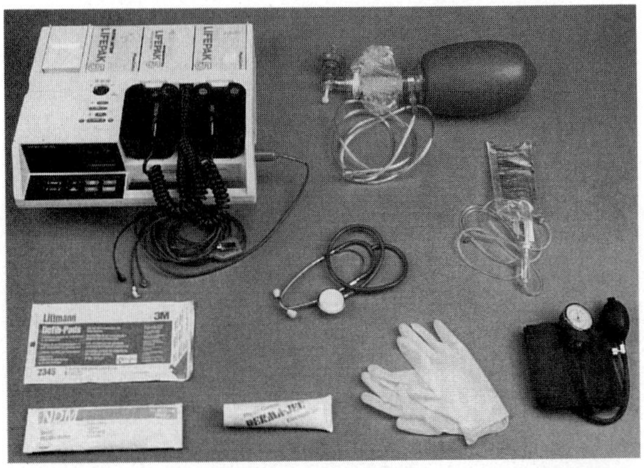

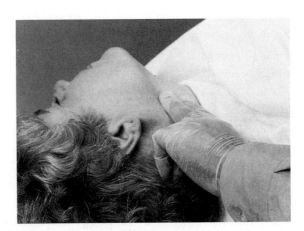

Figure 5-42 Equipment needed when performing vagal maneuvers.

Figure 5-43 Palpate carotid arteries.

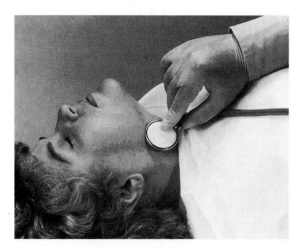

Figure 5-44 Auscultate for carotid bruits.

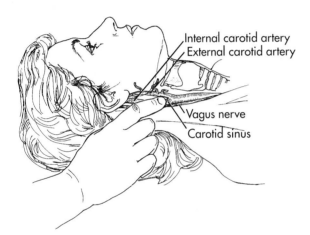

Figure 5-45 Anatomic landmarks for carotid sinus massage.

Internal carotid artery
External carotid artery
Vagus nerve
Carotid sinus

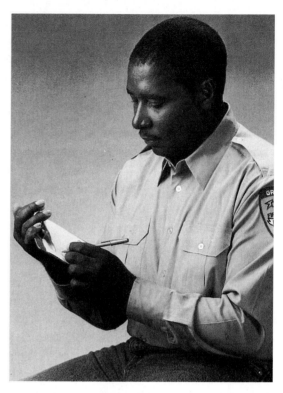

Figure 5-46 Document procedure, including EKG strip.

8. Use the flat side of two fingers and press firmly against the carotid artery toward the cervical vertebrae. You should be able to feel the pulse below your fingertips.

9. Massage the carotid sinus by using a circular motion.

10. Massage 60 to 120 seconds. Keep the monitor strip running to record the procedure and KEEP YOUR EYE ON THE MONITOR AT ALL TIMES.

11. Discontinue after 2 minutes, when the heart rate starts to slow, or when the patient experiences dizziness or a change in level of consciousness.

PEARLS & PITFALLS

Vagal Stimulation—Sometimes Things Just Don't Work Out!

◆ If vagal stimulation is unsuccessful in slowing or converting the tachydysrhythmia, synchronized cardioversion may be necessary.
◆ Increased parasympathetic tone may result in hypotension, nausea, vomiting, or bronchospasm.
◆ Rhythms that follow vagal stimulation, such as bradydysrhythmias or asystole, may require intervention.
◆ Syncope, hemiplegia, stroke or seizures may result as a result of cerebral complications.

12. If the procedure is unsuccessful on the right carotid, wait 2 to 3 minutes and repeat the procedure on the left side.

13. Report the results of the procedure to Medical Control.

14. Document the procedure, including a copy of the EKG strip (Figure 5-46).

◆ Noninvasive Pacing

Noninvasive pacing is the application of an external pacemaker for the emergency treatment of symptomatic bradycardia, heart block, or asystole until transvenous pacing can be initiated.

Indications
◆ Symptomatic bradycardia or heart block that causes decompensation of the patient (e.g., second- or third-degree block with associated hypotension, confusion, or chest pain)

Equipment
◆ EKG monitor
◆ EKG monitor leads
◆ BP cuff
◆ Stethoscope
◆ Pacemaker electrodes

Procedure
Not all noninvasive pacemakers are exactly alike. We are using a Lifepak 10. If your pacemaker differs from this one, consult the operator's manual supplied by the manufacturer for specifics.

1. Confirm the presence of the dysrhythmia and the patient's hemodynamic status.

2. Receive orders from Medical Control.

3. Explain the procedure to the patient (Figure 5-47).

4. Establish an IV if not already established.

5. Run an EKG strip to document the patient's rhythm. Label the strip with the patient's name, date, and time.

6. Adjust the EKG size so the machine can

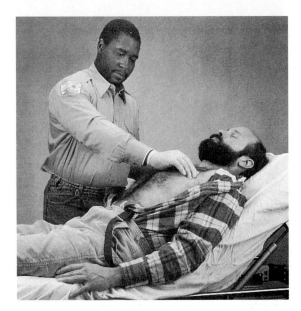

Figure 5-47 Explain the procedure to the patient.

sense the intrinsic QRS activity. The machine will then inhibit the pacing stimulus for the cycle (Figure 5-48).

7. Apply pacing electrodes in one of the following positions:

Anterior-posterior: This is the preferred placement. Place the negative electrode on left anterior chest, halfway between the xiphoid process and left nipple. The upper edge of the electrode should be below the nipple line (Figure 5-49). Place the positive electrode on the left posterior chest beneath the scapula and lateral to the spine (Figure 5-50). The placement of the electrodes affects current threshold.

Anterior-anterior: This position should be used only if the anterior-posterior position cannot be used. Place the negative electrode on the left chest, midaxillary over the fourth intercostal space. Place the positive electrode on the anterior right chest, subclavicular area.

8. Turn on the power.

9. Connect the pacing cable to the PACE connector on the right side of Lifepak 10.

10. Push the pacer button (Figure 5-51).

11. Select the desired pacing rate (Figure 5-52).

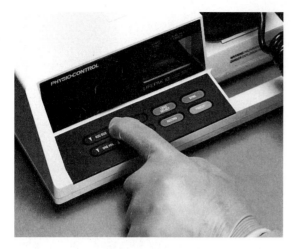

Figure 5-48   Adjust the EKG size.

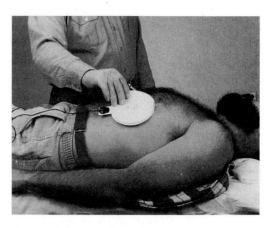

Figure 5-49   Apply the anterior pad.

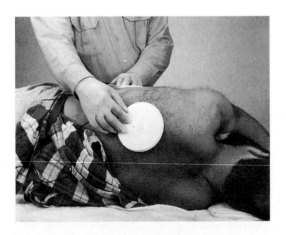

Figure 5-50   Apply the posterior pad.

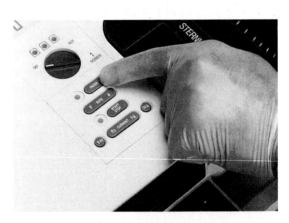

Figure 5-51   Depress the pacer button.

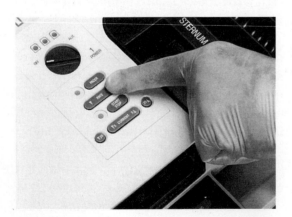

Figure 5-52   Select the appropriate heart rate.

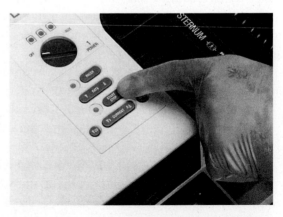

Figure 5-53   Depress the start/stop button to provide power to the pacer.

12. Observe the cardioscope for a "sense" marker on each QRS complex. If a "sense" marker is not present, readjust EKG size. If this fails, select another lead and readjust the size.

13. When the unit is sensing properly, activate the pacer by pushing START/STOP button. Pacer spikes should be seen with each pacer stimulus (Figure 5-53).

14. Increase the current slowly while observing the cardioscope for evidence of electrical pacing capture (Figure 5-54).

15. Assess for perfusion. Palpate the patient's pulse or check blood pressure (Figure 5-55).

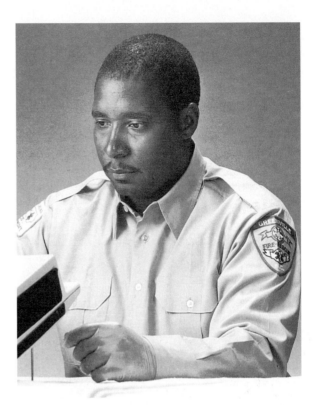

Figure 5-56 Observe the monitor.

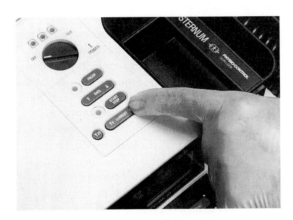

Figure 5-54 Increase current (mA) slowly, until capture occurs.

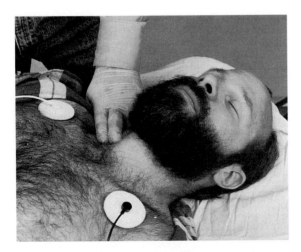

Figure 5-55 Check the patient's pulse.

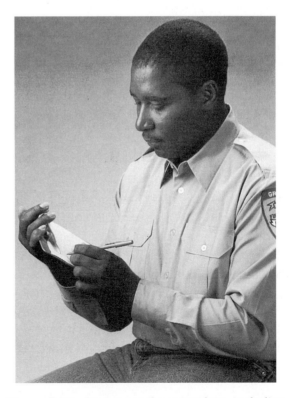

Figure 5-57 Document the procedure, including EKG strips.

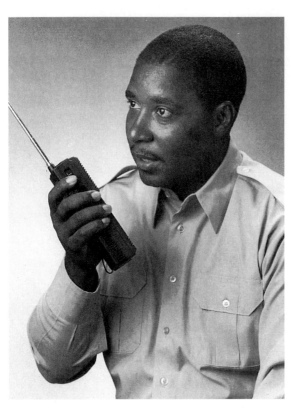

Figure 5-58 Advise Medical Control of the patient's status.

Noninvasive Cardiac Pacing

- Be sure the skin is dry and free of excess hair; however, do not shave the area or cleanse it with alcohol. If necessary, trim the hair with scissors. Prolonged pacing, especially at higher current levels, may result in skin irritation or burns under the electrodes. If this occurs, apply new electrodes and change the position slightly.
- Monitor through EKG leads rather than through the pacer leads or paddles.
- You should expect skeletal muscle contractions or twitching, but these are not an indication of pacing capture. Make sure to secure the patient's endotracheal tube and IVs to prevent displacement.
- Electrical capture is usually evidenced by a wide QRS and a tall broad T-wave, as well as a palpable pulse. Use the lowest current possible that produces capture to decrease the patient's discomfort. Sedation may be necessary in some patients.
- Monitor the patient's level of consciousness to evaluate brain perfusion.
- Generally you do not have to remove pacing electrodes to defibrillate because the position of the defibrillation paddles differs from that of the pacing electrodes.

16. Record EKG and document patient's rhythm, vital signs, and tolerance of pacing (Figures 5-56 and 5-57).

17. Report results to Medical Control (Figure 5-58).

Putting It All Together

The procedures discussed in this chapter on cardiac skills are of great importance to the paramedic. However, for most of these procedures to be successful, the paramedic must be sure that his equipment is ready for action. Dead batteries, torn EKG cables, or missing electrodes can put the patient's life in jeopardy. Routine procedures such as inventorying the unit or reconditioning the monitor/defibrillator batteries may save your patient's life.

Testing Your Knowledge

1. From the following list of EKG chest leads, select the one that provides the paramedic with the best picture of the heart's electrical activity.

   a. Lead I
   b. Lead II
   c. Lead III
   d. They all provide equal representation

2. The quick-look paddles allow the paramedic to rapidly ascertain ventricular fibrillation and consequently defibrillate the patient.

   a. True
   b. False

3. Excessive interference or artifact on the EKG monitor can result from all of the following EXCEPT:

   a. Dried gel on the electrode.
   b. Broken wire in the patient cable.
   c. Poor electrode contact.
   d. Defective heat stylus.

4. The random delivery of a high-intensity electrical charge to a fibrillating heart is known as:

   a. Defibrillation.
   b. Synchronized cardioversion.
   c. Unsynchronized countershock.
   d. a and c.

5. If your ambulance company does not possess pediatric defibrillator paddles, you will be unable to countershock any pediatric patients under the age of 12.

   a. True
   b. False

6. From the following list, select the correct joule setting to initially defibrillate a 44-lb child.

   a. 20 J
   b. 30 J
   c. 40 J
   d. 50 J

7. Synchronized cardioversion is designed to interrupt an ectopic pacemaker by monitoring the rhythm for which wave of the EKG?

   a. P-wave
   b. Q-wave
   c. R-wave
   d. T-wave

8. List the two most commonly used forms of vagal maneuver used in the prehospital setting.

9. Even with a properly performed vagal maneuver, the patient may experience bradycardia, asystole, or cerebrovascular accident.

   a. True
   b. False

10. Noninvasive cardiac pacing is recommended in all of the following dysrhythmias EXCEPT:

   a. Ventricular fibrillation.
   b. Asystole.
   c. Third-degree heart block.
   d. Sinus bradycardia with hypotension.

11. Electrical capture of a noninvasive cardiac pacemaker is usually represented on an EKG by a narrow QRS complex and short T-wave.

   a. True
   b. False

Answers are in Appendix A.

BIBLIOGRAPHY

Budassi S, Barber J: *Mosby's manual of emergency care: Practice and Procedures,* ed 2, St. Louis, 1984, Mosby.

California Emergency Care: *Student handbook EMT-P skills test,* ed 4, Lafayette, Calif, 1983, California Emergency Care Standards and Training.

Caroline N: *Emergency care in the streets,* ed 3, Boston, 1987, Little, Brown.

Application of EKG Monitor Leads

Procedure	Possible points	Points awarded
Explain procedure to patient.	1	
Peel off backing from electrode.	1	
Identify anatomic landmarks.	1	
Apply electrodes.	1	
Attach monitor cables to electrodes.	1	
Connect leads to monitor.	1	
Turn monitor to "on" position and select proper lead.	2	
Adjust EKG to desired height.	1	
Adjust QRS volume.	1	
Depress record button and run minimum of 6-second strip.	1	
Label EKG strip with patient's name, date, and time.	1	
TOTAL POINTS	**12**	

COMMENTS _____

_____

_____

Quick-Look Paddles

Quick-look paddles are used in the initial phase of cardiac arrest, before the patient is connected to traditional EKG leads.

Procedure	Possible points	Points awarded
Confirm pulselessness and breathlessness.	2	
Initiate CPR until paddles are prepared.	1	
Turn monitor/defibrillator to "on" position.	1	
Turn lead selector to PADDLES.	1	
Apply defibrillation pads to patient's chest or apply conductive gel to paddles.	1	
Place paddles firmly on chest in proper location.	1	
Adjust EKG size to desired height.	1	
Observe scope and determine rhythm.	1	
Check pulse and verify pulselessness.	1	
If potentially fatal ventricular dysrhythmia is noted, set energy level to appropriate level and charge paddles.	2	
Verbally and visually "clear" area.	1	
Depress both paddle buttons simultaneously.	1	
Check scope for change in rhythm and check for pulse.	2	
Repeat shocks two additional times, provided there is no change in rhythm.	2	
Connect patient to three-lead monitoring.	1	
Document event, including EKG strips.	1	
TOTAL POINTS	**20**	

COMMENTS

Defibrillation

Defibrillation, or unsynchronized countershock, is the random delivery of a high-intensity electrical charge to the heart. (This skill sheet assumes that the quick-look procedure is complete and that the patient is connected to three-lead monitoring.)

Procedure	Possible points	Points awarded
Observe scope and determine rhythm.	1	
Check pulse and verify pulselessness.	1	
If potentially fatal ventricular dysrhythmia is noted, set energy level to appropriate level and charge paddles.	2	
Apply defibrillation pads to patient's chest or apply conductive gel to paddles.	1	
Place paddles firmly on chest in proper location.	1	
Verbally and visually "clear" area.	1	
Depress both paddle buttons simultaneously.	1	
Check scope for change in rhythm and check for pulse.	2	
Document event, including EKG strips.	1	
TOTAL POINTS	**11**	

COMMENTS _____

_____

_____

Synchronized Cardioversion

Synchronized cardioversion is the timed delivery of an electrical shock to the heart. This shock is designed to interrupt an ectopic pacemaker so that the sinus node can regain control.

Procedure	Possible points	Points awarded
Confirm presence of dysrhythmia and patient's hemodynamic status, including a copy of the EKG strip.	2	
Explain procedure to patient.	1	
Establish IV, if not already performed.	1	
Premedicate patient, if needed.	1	
Turn monitor/defibrillator to "on" position and select proper lead.	2	
Depress "sync" button.	1	
Verify that R-waves are of appropriate height to be monitored.	1	
Select joule setting.	1	
Apply defibrillator pads to patient's chest or apply conductive gel to paddles.	1	
Push charge buttons. Verify that synchronizer is "marking" R-waves.	2	
Turn on EKG paper recorder.	1	
Place paddles firmly on chest in proper location.	1	
Verbally and visually "clear" area.	1	
Depress both paddle buttons simultaneously and wait for shock to occur.	1	
Evaluate patient.	1	
Document procedure.	1	
TOTAL POINTS	**19**	

COMMENTS

Vagal Maneuvers

Vagal maneuvers stimulate the vagus nerve in an effort to cause a slowing of the heart rate. They are used in the prehospital setting in the treatment of supraventricular tachycardias. Either Valsalva's maneuver or carotid sinus massage is acceptable in this exercise.

Procedure	Possible points	Points awarded
Confirm presence of dysrhythmia and patient's hemodynamic status, including copy of EKG strip.	2	
Explain procedure to patient.	1	
Establish IV, if not already performed.	1	
Prepare all ACLS equipment.	1	
Place patient in supine position with the head hyperextended.	1	
Check equality of carotid pulses—palpate separately.	1	
Auscultate carotid pulses for bruits.	1	
Turn patient's head slightly to left and relocate carotid pulse.	1	
Use flat side of two fingers and press firmly against the carotid artery. Massage carotid sinus with slow, circular motion.	1	
Evaluate EKG during entire process and stop process with conversion of rhythm.	1	
Evaluate patient and provide supportive care.	1	
Document procedure.	1	
TOTAL POINTS	**13**	

COMMENTS _____

_____

_____

Noninvasive Cardiac Pacing

Noninvasive cardiac pacing is the application of an external pacemaker for the emergency treatment of symptomatic bradycardia, heart block, or asystole.

Procedure	Possible points	Points awarded
Confirm presence of dysrhythmia and patient's hemodynamic status, including copy of EKG strip.	2	
Explain procedure to patient.	1	
Establish IV, if not already performed.	1	
Adjust EKG size so machine can sense intrinsic QRS activity.	1	
Apply pacemaker electrodes, using either the anterior-posterior or anterior-anterior approach.	1	
Turn monitor/defibrillator to "on" position and select proper lead.	1	
Plug pacing cable into connector.	1	
Select desired pacing rate.	1	
Observe cardioscope for a "sense" marker on each QRS complex. If not present, increase QRS size.	1	
Once sensing, depress "start" button and observe for pacer spikes.	1	
Increase current (mA) slowly while observing for evidence of electrical capture.	1	
Assess patient's perfusion.	1	
Record EKG and document procedure.	1	
TOTAL POINTS	**14**	

COMMENTS _____

_____

_____

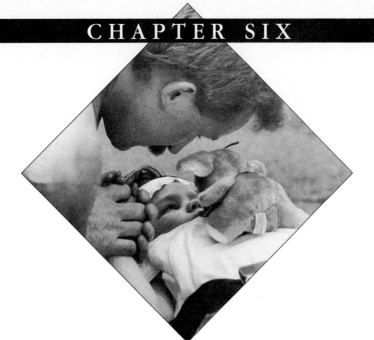

CHAPTER SIX

Advanced Pediatric Skills

Objectives

A paramedic should be able to:

1. Explain the rationale for performing a toe-to-head survey on a pediatric patient.

2. Explain how heart rate, respiratory rate, and blood pressure change as a child matures.

3. Select the appropriate-size endotracheal tube (ETT) for children of different ages.

4. List two situations in which using digital intubation would be appropriate.

5. List two situations in which using oral intubation would be appropriate.

6. List four anatomic differences between pediatric and adult airways.

7. Given a picture, identify the anatomic landmarks for venous catheterization of the umbilicus.

8. Given the appropriate mannequins, perform the following pediatric skills:
   a. Oral laryngoscopy and intubation
   b. Digital intubation
   c. Peripheral intravenous access
   d. Scalp vein access
   e. Intraosseous access
   f. Umbilical catheterization

Photo courtesy *San Diego Union Tribune*/Robert Gauthier.

Case Scenario

"Paramedic Unit 3, respond to 4323 Barrington Road, a small child experiencing difficulty breathing." On arrival, you are met by a frantic mother who is screaming that her son has choked on a hot dog.

A 4-year-old boy is lying on the kitchen floor where the father is performing backblows and chest thrusts. The child is markedly cyanotic and appears to be moving no air. Ventilation attempts are unsuccessful. You perform direct laryngoscopy and remove a large chunk of meat from the airway, using McGill forceps. Occasional spontaneous respirations resume, and you note some improvement in color after bagging the child with a bag-valve-mask (BVM) and supplemental oxygen. The heart rate is weak and bradycardic. The patient responds inappropriately to painful stimuli.

You perform endotracheal intubation via direct laryngoscopy to enhance oxygenation. Sinus rhythm is shown on the EKG monitor at a rate of 110 beats per minute. During transport an intravenous line (IV) of lactated Ringer's is initiated in the right saphenous vein, using a 20-gauge catheter. The child becomes more alert throughout transport. After 3 days in the hospital, the patient is released.

The pediatric patient is considered by many prehospital care providers as one of the most physically and emotionally challenging of all Emergency Medical Service (EMS) calls. Many things that are not factors in adults demand attention in children. The patient's developmental age, weight, and mental status can greatly affect assessment and treatment. More difficult for many paramedics, however, is the emotional stress associated with the critical pediatric call. In many cases, a paramedic who has a child near the same age or size may associate the patient with his or her own child. Critical incident stress debriefing is recommended for any paramedic following a serious pediatric emergency.

It is interesting to note that the majority of pediatric EMS calls are traumatic, whereas medical emergencies comprise the bulk of adult responses. Being called to the scene of an injured or ill child, especially an infant, challenges even the most experienced paramedic. Although the priorities of airway, breathing, circulation, and disability are the same as for any patient, many other aspects are different.

The customary approach of introducing oneself and asking, "How may I help you?" does not work with a 2-year-old. Often the child is unable or unwilling to talk with paramedics, and the perception of parents or bystanders must be relied on. Physical findings are quite different from those found in adults. In addition to the obvious size difference, vital signs change as children grow. The needs of the parents, as well as the child, must be addressed. The paramedic must be calm, controlled, and competent with each pediatric situation, with both the child and the parent.

◆ Patient Evaluation

The evaluation of the pediatric patient may vary from that of the adult. As noted in the introduction, communication is not always optimal with a young child. Developmental characteristics play an important role in the evaluation of any patient under the age of 18 years. The ability to speak, the willingness to cooperate, and the feeling of independence greatly affect a paramedic's role in gathering information. Especially with young children who do not verbalize well, observation is a key skill for the prehospital care provider. For example, rubbing an area can often indicate pain or infection; fever and a high-pitched scream can be a sign of meningitis. The parent's observations are also very important and should be considered and documented in all cases.

Physical examination is often more successful in the preschooler or younger patient when performed in a toe-to-head sequence, rather than the traditional head-to-toe. This technique

Table 6-1 Normal Vital Signs

Age	Respiratory rate	Heart rate	Systolic blood pressure
Newborn	30-50	120-160	50-70
Infant (1-12 months)	20-30	80-140	70-100
Toddler (1-3 years)	20-30	80-130	80-110
Preschooler (3-5 years)	20-30	80-120	80-110
School Age (6-12 years)	20-30	70-110	80-120
Adolescent (13+ years)	12-20	55-105	100-120

From Eichelberger MR, Ball JW, Pratsch GS, et al: *Pediatric emergencies*, ed 1, Englewood Cliffs, NJ, 1992, Brady (Prentice-Hall).

allows a paramedic to evaluate the legs and chest before examining the head and facial area. Looking into the child's mouth, ears, and eyes often causes crying, which makes auscultation of the chest and any further examination very difficult.

Remember, children are not small adults and cannot be evaluated as such. Vital signs vary greatly according to the developmental age and size of the child. Table 6-1 summarizes the variations in pulse, respiration, and blood pressure according to age.

In addition to using the guidelines in Table 6-1, various formulas exist for estimating vital signs and weights for pediatrics. For example, to estimate the systolic blood pressure for any child over the age of 1 year, the following formula can be used:

80 + (two times the child's age in years)

Thus the expected systolic blood pressure of a 7-year-old would be 80 + (2 × 7) = 94.

The weight of a child can be estimated using a similar formula. To approximate the normal weight in kilograms, the following equation is suggested:

8 + (two times the child's age in years)

Thus the same 7-year-old above should weigh 8 + (2 × 7) = 22 kg. This formula is extremely useful when administering pediatric medications.

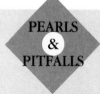

Pediatric Equipment

Unfortunately, adult equipment does not always fit pediatric patients. It is important to have the right equipment to do the right job. This is especially true for airway and ventilation equipment, blood pressure cuffs, and defibrillation paddles.

Pediatric intravenous equipment and medications are necessities in the provision of advanced life support for children. I/O needles, small-gauge catheters, and prefilled pediatric drugs save time and allow for more efficient care to the small patient.

◆ Pediatric Laryngoscopy and Oral Endotracheal Intubation

Laryngoscopy is the procedure used for visualizing the upper airway using a device called a laryngoscope. The laryngoscope allows for direct access to the glottic opening by lifting the tongue and mandible. Endotracheal intubation is the process of placing an open-ended tube into the trachea to secure the airway and improve ventilation.

Background

Controlling the airway is the most crucial skill in the assessment and management of any patient. However, this is especially true for pediatrics. Unlike adults, who often require total resuscitation efforts, many pediatric patients rapidly respond with aggressive ventilation and oxygenation. Each ventilation should be given gently, and just enough should be given to accomplish chest rise. High-pressured blasts of air, such as those given with a demand-valve resuscitator, are apt to cause pleural injury. A bag-valve resuscitator should be used, since chest compliance can be easily felt by the paramedic squeezing the bag.

Endotracheal intubation provides the most secure airway in the prehospital setting. The pediatric airway is anatomically different from that of the adult and thus requires special handling and equipment. Some of the anatomic differences include:

- A head that is relatively larger than the neck and torso.
- A small face with a relatively flat nasal bridge.
- A relatively large tongue in relation to the mouth.
- A larynx that is located more anterior and at the level of the cricoid cartilage.
- An airway whose smallest diameter is subglottic.

Indications

- In any child who is unable to protect his own airway
- Ineffective BVM ventilation
- Tracheal suctioning of the neonate for meconium aspiration

Contraindications

- There are no contraindications for intubation of the pediatric patient. However, special precaution should be taken with the traumatized patient. Cervical alignment must be maintained during laryngoscopy and tube placement.

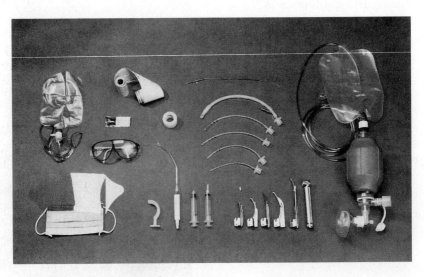

Figure 6-1 Intubation equipment.

Equipment (Figure 6-1)

- Suction device with appropriate size catheters and bulb syringes
- Oxygen
- Pediatric BVM with reservoir bag
- Laryngoscope handle and variety of pediatric blades (sizes 0, 1, 2)
- Spare laryngoscope light bulbs
- ETTs (2.5 to 6.5 mm)
- 10-ml syringe
- Water-soluble lubricant
- 1-inch tape
- Pediatric stylet
- Gloves
- Eye protection (goggles)

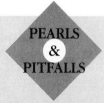

PEARLS
&
PITFALLS

Intubation Equipment

The anatomic differences in the pediatric airway require a paramedic to use equipment, most notably the ETT, that is slightly different from that used when intubating the adult. An ETT the approximate size of the patient's little finger is suggested. Up to the age of 8 years, the airway is narrowest at the cricoid ring, rather than at the vocal cords. This narrowing serves to seal the airway around the ETT, so that a cuff is not necessary. In fact, use of a cuffed tube in this age group may result in damage to the trachea (Table 6-2).

Generally, Miller blades are used in children, since they allow for better visualization of the airway. This is a result of the anterior and high positioning of the larynx. Other comparable blades may be used as guided by local protocol (Table 6-3).

Table 6-2	Tube Sizes for Pediatric Intubation	
Age	Endotracheal tube (mm)	Suction catheter
Premature	2.5	6F
Newborn	3.0	6F
6 month	3.5	8F
18 month	4.0	8F
3 years	4.5	8F
5 years	5.0	10F
6 years	5.5	10F
8 years	6.0	10F
12 years	6.5	10F

From EMT-Paramedic—National Standard Curriculum: Washington, DC, 1985, US Dept of Transportation, US Government Printing Office.

Table 6-3	Blade Sizes for Pediatric Intubation
Age	Blade size
Premature	No. 0 straight Miller
Term newborn to 3-year old	No. 1 straight Miller
3-year old to adolescent	No. 2 straight Miller or curved Macintosh
Adolescent	No. 3 curved Macintosh

From EMT-Paramedic—National Standard Curriculum: Washington, DC, 1985, US Dept. of Transportation, US Government Printing Office.

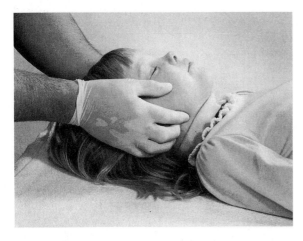

Figure 6-2   Position the head and hyperventilate the patient.

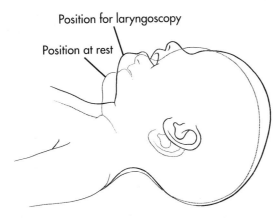

Position for laryngoscopy

Position at rest

Figure 6-3   Position the head at rest; for laryngoscopy.

Procedure

1. Observe universal precautions (gloves and eye protection).

2. Position the head (Figure 6-2) and hyperventilate the patient with a BVM and high-concentration oxygen. Because of the relatively large head size, some flexion of the head may naturally occur (Figure 6-3). It may be necessary to extend the head slightly so that the face looks straight up and provides an open airway.

3. Select and check the proper equipment. (See Tables 6-2 and 6-3 for suggested blade and tube sizes.) Insert stylet into the ETT and lubricate the tube with water-soluble jelly. It may be necessary to lubricate the stylet slightly to advance it into the lumen of the tube.

4. Reposition the nontraumatized child by placing a small towel under the shoulders (Figure 6-4). This position facilitates visualization of the airway because of the anatomic differences.

5. Holding the laryngoscope in your left hand, introduce the laryngoscope into the right side of the child's mouth (Figure 6-5). Sweep

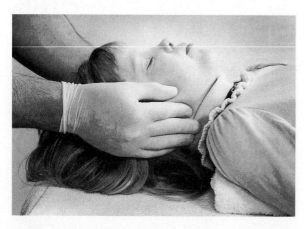

Figure 6-4   Reposition the nontraumatized patient by placing a small towel under the shoulders.

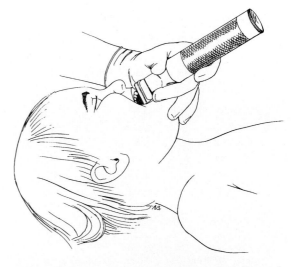

Figure 6-5   Hold the laryngoscope handle with your left hand and enter the right side of the mouth.

the tongue to the left side and simultaneously lift the chin forward. Expose the vocal cords by lifting the epiglottis with the tip of the Miller blade (Figure 6-6). Be careful not to advance the blade too far and accidentally lacerate the vocal cords.

6. Gently insert the ETT until you see the tip of the tube advance past the glottic opening (Figure 6-7, *A* and *B*).

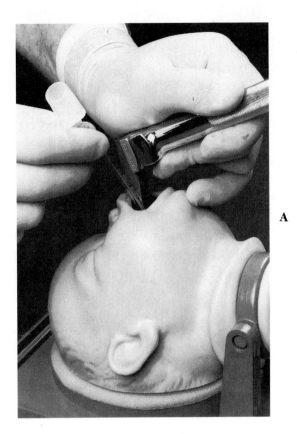

A

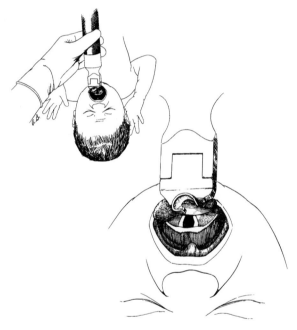

Figure 6-6 Expose the vocal cords by lifting the epiglottis with a straight blade.

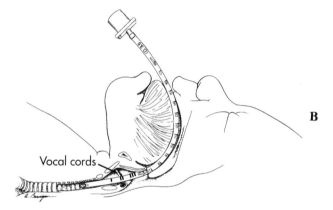

B

Vocal cords

Figure 6-7 **A** and **B**, Correct placement of a non-cuffed ETT.

7. Remove the laryngoscope blade and stylet, while tightly holding the tube in place with your right hand.

8. Ventilate the patient using a BVM and watch for chest rise. Confirm placement by auscultating the chest bilaterally and the epigastrium with a stethoscope (Figure 6-8, *A* and *B*). (Adjuncts such as end-tidal carbon dioxide detectors can be used if approved by the local jurisdiction).

9. Secure the tube, using tape.

10. Reassess tube placement after taping. Be aware that any substantial movement may result in displacement of the tube. Reassess often.

PEARLS & PITFALLS

Reflex Bradycardia

During laryngoscopy the child is not receiving ventilation or supplemental oxygen. Thus, hyperventilation should always precede intubation attempts, and the heart rate should be monitored. When children experience marked oxygen deprivation, they develop a condition known as reflex bradycardia. If the heart rate slows down to less than 80 beats per minute, remove the laryngoscope immediately and hyperventilate the patient for 2 minutes.

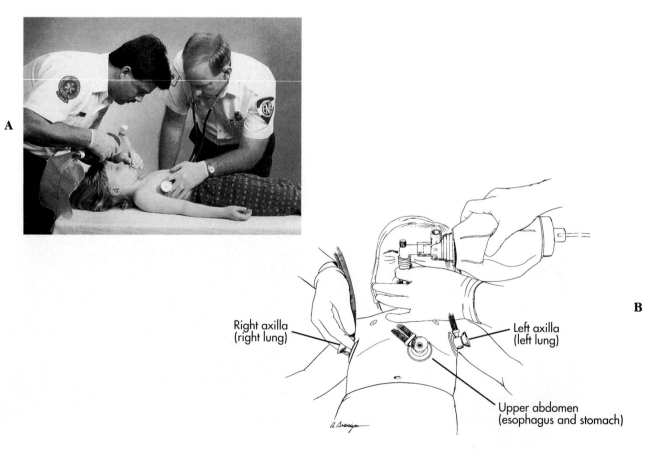

Right axilla (right lung)

Left axilla (left lung)

Upper abdomen (esophagus and stomach)

Figure 6-8 **A** and **B**, Confirm placement by listening to the chest and epigastrium.

◆ Digital Endotracheal Intubation

Digital endotracheal intubation is a blind procedure that positions an ETT into the trachea without the aid of a laryngoscope. It is accomplished by placing the ETT into the pharynx of the patient with the paramedic directing the tube into the glottic opening, using the tip of the middle finger.

Background

Special pediatric situations occur that require a paramedic to use skills that are seldom performed in the prehospital setting. Digital intubation is one of those special occasions. Anatomic differences and injuries involving the pediatric airway often make traditional endotracheal intubation attempts futile.

Indications

- Inability to successfully place an ETT using a laryngoscope and blade
- Severe facial trauma that prohibits visualization of the vocal cords
- Mechanism of injury or signs indicating a possible cervical neck injury in which traditional intubation techniques may be detrimental to the patient

Contraindications

- There are essentially no contraindications to digital intubation. However, precaution must be used when intubating the patient with a possible cervical injury. Neutral cervical alignment must be maintained throughout the procedure. The child should be unresponsive before attempting the procedure.

Equipment

- Suction device
- Oxygen
- Pediatric BVM with reservoir bag
- Laryngoscope and appropriate-size blades
- ETTs (2.5 to 6.5)
- 10-ml syringe
- Water-soluble lubricant
- 1-inch tape
- Pediatric stylet
- Gloves
- Eye protection

Procedure

1. Observe universal precautions.

2. Position the head and hyperventilate the patient with a BVM and high-concentration oxygen (Figure 6-9). Because of the relatively large head size, some flexion of the head may naturally occur. It may be necessary to extend the head slightly so that the face looks straight up and provides an open airway.

3. Select and check the proper equipment. (See Table 6-2 for suggested tube size.) Insert the stylet into the ETT and lubricate the tube with water-soluble jelly. It may be necessary to lubricate the stylet slightly to advance it into the lumen of the tube.

4. Reposition the child by placing a small towel under the shoulders. This position will facilitate proper anatomic alignment of the airway. (This step may be skipped if there is reason to suspect spinal injury.)

5. Position yourself so that you are facing the child and the palm of your hand rests on the child's chin (Figure 6-10).

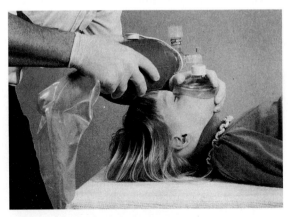

Figure 6-9 Hyperventilate the patient with a BVM and high-concentration oxygen.

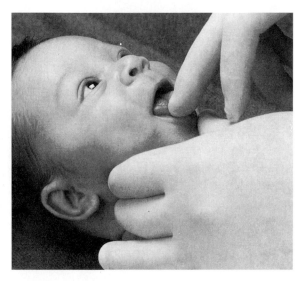

Figure 6-10 Position yourself facing the patient. Lift the epiglottis with the middle finger.

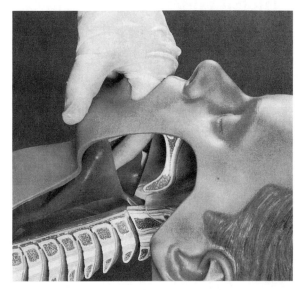

Figure 6-11 Lift the epiglottis with the middle finger.

6. With the middle finger, reach into the oropharynx and feel for the epiglottis. Once located, lift the epiglottis anteriorly (Figure 6-11).

7. Introduce the ETT into the oropharynx and supraglottic area.

8. With your middle finger, identify the tip of the tube and place your finger posterior to the tube (Figure 6-12).

9. Simultaneously advance the tube while positioning it anteriorly toward the glottic opening. Slide the tube through the cords.

10. Remove your finger and hold the tube with one hand, while applying a BVM with the other. Ventilate the child and watch for chest rise. Confirm placement by auscultating the chest and epigastrium with a stethoscope (Figure 6-13). (If the child is over 8 years of age, a cuffed ETT may be appropriate. In these cases, inflation of the cuff would be performed in this step).

11. Secure the tube using tape.

12. Reassess tube placement after taping. Be aware that any substantial movement may result in displacement of the tube. Reassess often.

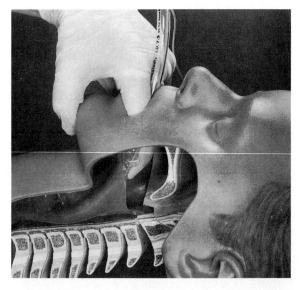

Figure 6-12 Position the tube into the glottic opening.

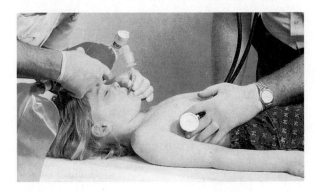

Figure 6-13 Confirm tube placement.

Vascular Access

Vascular access is the procedure of gaining entry into the circulatory system via artery, vein, or intramedullary cavity. In the prehospital setting, a paramedic is limited to the latter two routes. Hence, we will discuss only those procedures.

Background

Although airway and ventilatory problems assume the highest priority in pediatric emergencies, there is often a need for vascular access once the airway has been addressed. As with adults, intravenous access is necessary for two reasons: to administer crystalloid fluids for volume expansion, and to provide an IV for the administration of medications (Table 6-4).

Special equipment is often used in the initiation of the pediatric IV that is not used in the adult patient. For example, smaller gauge over-the-needle catheters (Nos. 20, 22, or 24) are used, as well as butterfly needles. Specially designed intraosseous needles or spinal needles are used for boring through the tibia to access the marrow of the intramedullary cavity. Umbilical catheters are used in the neonate when accessing the umbilical vein.

Pediatric fluid administration must be carefully regulated. In all cases a microdrip solution set should be used. Optimally, the use of a volume-control device (such as the Buretrol shown in Figure 6-14) is strongly rec-

Table 6-4 Drugs Used in ACLS for Infants and Children

Drug	Dose	How supplied	Remarks
Atropine sulfate	0.01-0.03 mg/kg	0.1 mg/ml	IV fast push
Calcium chloride	20 mg/kg	100 mg/ml (10%)	IV slow push
Dopamine hydrochloride	2-10 μg/kg/min.	200 mg/5ml	Alpha receptor dominate at ≥10 mg/kg/min—titrate to effect
Epinephrine	0.01 mg/kg	1:10,000 (1 mg/10 ml)	1:1000 must be diluted
Epinephrine infusion	Start at 0.1 mg/kg/min	1:1000 (1 mg)	Usual effect infusion less than 1.5 mg/kg/min
Furosemide	1 mg/kg	10 mg/ml	IV Slow—every 2 hours
Isoproterenol hydrochloride	Start at 0.1 μg/kg/min.	1 mg/5 ml	Usual effect 0.1-1 mg/kg/min—titrate to effect
Lidocaine	1 mg/kg/dose	10 mg/ml (1%) 20 mg/ml (2%)	IV slow push
Lidocaine infusion	0.02-0.03 mg/kg/min.	10 mg/ml (1%) 20 mg/ml (2%) 40 mg/ml (4%)	Start at 20 μg/kg/min—titrate up to 30 μg/kg/min
Naloxone hydrochloride	0.01 mg/kg 10 μg/kg neonatal	0.4 mg/ml 0.02 mg/ml	Repeat every 3-5 minutes as needed; Darvon overdose may require 0.1 mg/kg
Sodium bicarbonate	1-2 mEq/kg	1 mEq/ml	Repeat dose in 10 minutes or by ABGs

From EMT-Paramedic—National Standard Curriculum: Washington, DC, 1985, US Dept of Transportation, US Government Printing Office.

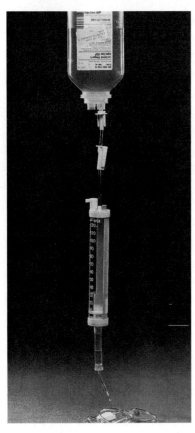

Figure 6-14   Buretrol volume–control solution set.

ommended to prevent accidental fluid overload.

◆ Peripheral Vein Access

Background

Peripheral access in the neonate or pediatric patient can be very challenging, even for an experienced paramedic. The small size of the vessel, along with a child who is often uncooperative, can make this procedure very difficult. It is important to select a catheter that is not too large for the vein. Generally, the large veins of the arm, leg, or scalp are selected, using a 20-, 22- or 24-gauge over-the-needle catheter. The external jugular vein is very difficult to access because of the short neck on a child and is often not attempted.

Indications

* Any medical condition, such as cardiopulmonary arrest, accidental overdose, or sepsis, that suggests an IV or possible medication administration
* Any traumatic condition such as head injury, multiple fractures, or shock that suggests the need for volume resuscitation

Contraindications

* There are no contraindications to initiating an IV in the pediatric patient who is in need of vascular access.

Equipment (Figure 6-15)

* Crystalloid intravenous solution
* Intravenous solution set (microdrip or Buretrol-type)
* Alcohol or povidone-iodine preps
* Tourniquet or rubber band
* 20-, 22-, or 24-gauge over-the-needle catheter or butterfly needle
* 1/2-inch or 1-inch hypoallergenic tape
* Armboard (if needed)

Procedure for an Extremity Venipuncture

1. Observe universal precautions (gloves and eye protection).

2. Assemble the necessary equipment. Set up intravenous solution, flush tubing, and tear tape.

3. Immobilize the extremity, if necessary.

4. Place a venous tourniquet proximal to the proposed site. A rubber band can be used if the extremity is very small (Figure 6-16).

5. Locate a suitable vein that will accept a catheter. Cleanse the site, using an alcohol or povidone-iodine prep (Figure 6-17).

6. Perform venipuncture, using correct, aseptic technique. Watch for blood return. Because of the small catheter lumen and lower venous pressure, the flashback may not be as apparent as it is in adults (Figure 6-18).

7. Slowly advance the catheter and remove the needle.

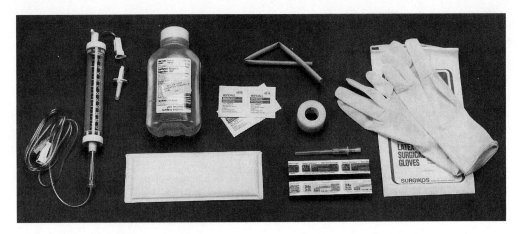

Figure 6-15 Equipment for peripheral vein access.

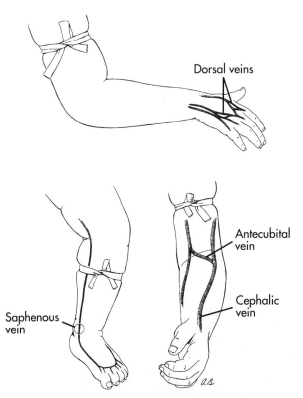

Figure 6-16 Place a venous tourniquet proximal to the proposed IV site.

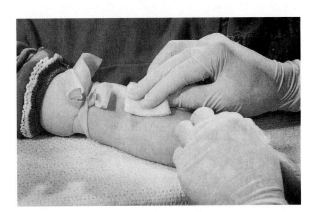

Figure 6-17 Cleanse the site.

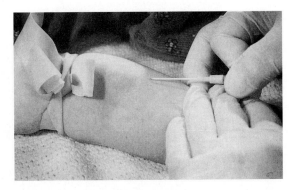

Figure 6-18 Flashbacks are not always apparent.

8. Release the tourniquet and attach intravenous solution.

9. Slowly introduce fluid into the vein. If patent, adjust flow rate.

10. Secure the catheter, using an acceptable taping method. With an active child, extra tape or roller-gauze dressing is advisable (Figure 6-19).

11. Routinely reconfirm IV patency and drip rate (Figure 6-20).

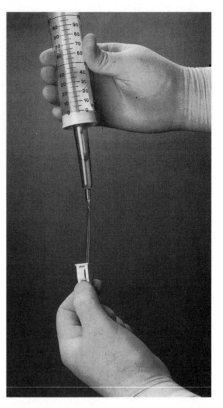

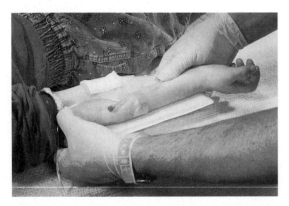

Figure 6-19 Secure the IV with tape and an armboard.

Figure 6-20 Confirm IV patency and drip rate.

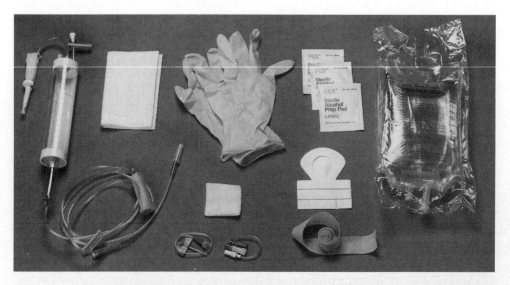

Figure 6-21 Assemble the necessary equipment.

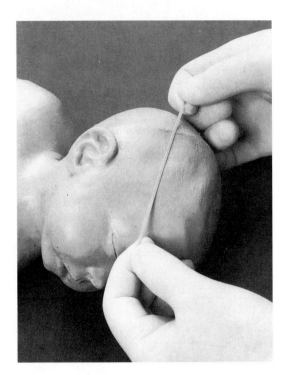

Figure 6-22   Place a rubber band tourniquet around the head.

Procedure for a Scalp Vein Venipuncture

1. Observe universal precautions (gloves and eye protection).

2. Assemble the necessary equipment. Set up intravenous solution, flush tubing, and tear tape (Figure 6-21).

3. Immobilize the child on a pediatric spineboard or immobilization device, if necessary.

4. Place a rubber band tourniquet around the head (Figure 6-22).

5. Locate a suitable vein that will accept a catheter. Cleanse the site, using an alcohol or povidone-iodine prep. It may be necessary to shave a small area of hair.

6. Perform venipuncture using correct, aseptic technique (Figure 6-23, *A* and *B*). Watch for blood return. Because of the small catheter lumen and lower venous pressure, the flashback may not be as apparent as it is in adults. In many cases, a small-gauge butterfly needle is used in initiating the scalp vein IV.

7. Slowly advance the catheter and remove the needle, if using an over-the-needle catheter. If using a butterfly, slowly advance the needle.

8. Release the tourniquet and attach intravenous solution (Figure 6-24).

9. Slowly introduce fluid into the vein. If patent, adjust flow rate.

10. Secure the catheter or needle, using an acceptable taping method. With an active

A
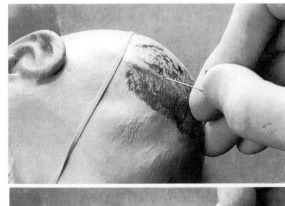

B
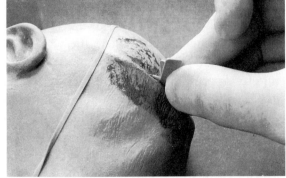

Figure 6-23   **A** and **B**, Perform careful venipuncture.

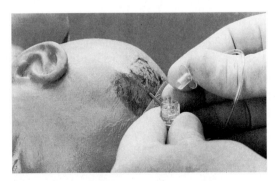

Figure 6-24   Release the tourniquet and attach IV tubing.

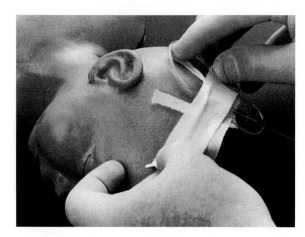

Figure 6-25 Tape securely.

child, extra tape or roller-gauze dressing may be advisable (Figure 6-25).

11. Routinely reconfirm IV patency and drip rate.

◆ Umbilical Vein Catheterization

Umbilical vein catheterization (UVC) is the process of gaining intravenous access by placing a specialized catheter or tubing into the umbilical vein of the neonatal umbilicus.

Background

UVC is making its way into the field setting. This procedure allows a paramedic to administer fluids or medications when percutaneous cannulation into a small vein is technically impossible.

The umbilical vein catheter is not without serious risks. Local and systemic infection, thrombus formation, and possible emboli are all potential side effects. In addition, too aggressive or poor placement by the paramedic may result in the tip of the catheter entering the portal system of the liver.

Indication

◆ Neonatal patient in need of IV access, but does not have accessible peripheral veins.

Contraindications

◆ There are no significant contraindications, especially when used in a life-threatening illness or injury.

Equipment (Figure 6-26)

◆ Sterile scalpel
◆ Umbilical tape
◆ Two sterile, delicately curved 5-inch hemostats
◆ Sterile gauze pads (4 × 4)
◆ No. 3.5, 5, or 7 Fr. umbilical catheter
◆ Luer-Lok disposable stopcock
◆ Sterile scissors
◆ Povidone-iodine swabs
◆ Intravenous solution
◆ Microdrip or Buretrol-type solution set
◆ Heparin (concentration of 10 U/1 ml of fluid)
◆ Gloves
◆ Eye protection (goggles)
◆ Sterile drapes

Procedure

1. Observe universal precautions.

2. Prepare the above equipment.

3. Restrain the infant, if necessary.

4. Clean and drape the area. The umbilicus should be cleansed, using povidone-iodine solution (Figure 6-27).

5. Place a loose tie of umbilical tape around the base of the umbilicus.

6. Identify one of the two umbilical veins (Figure 6-28).

7. Using a sterile hemostat, insert the tip of the hemostat into the lumen of the vein. Gently open the hemostat to dilate the vessel.

8. Introduce and advance the umbilical catheter approximately 3 to 4 inches (Figure 6-29). This will place the catheter into the inferior vena cava of the infant. You should note blood return after inserting the catheter. Do not force the catheter because you may cause severe hemorrhage or liver injury.

9. Hook up the catheter to a three-way

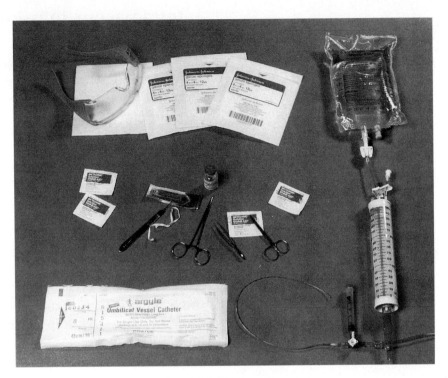

Figure 6-26 UVC equipment.

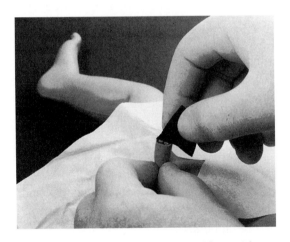

Figure 6-27 Cleanse the area with povidone-iodine solution.

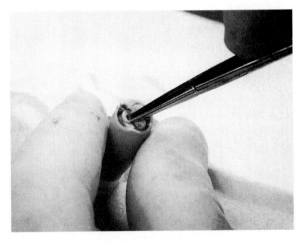

Figure 6-28 Identify one of the two umbilical veins.

stopcock. Flush the catheter with 1 ml of heparin solution (Figure 6-30).

10. Secure the catheter, using the piece of umbilical tape, by tying the tape around the umbilicus (Figure 6-31).

11. After securing the catheter, hook the IV tubing to the stopcock to allow for the administration of fluids and/or medications.

12. Monitor the umbilicus for bleeding. A dressing is usually not used in this situation so that the umbilicus can be viewed.

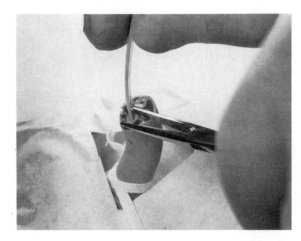

Figure 6-29 Advance the catheter approximately 3 to 4 inches.

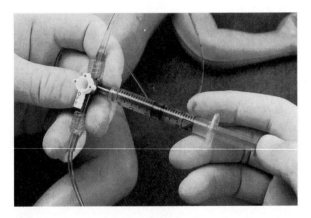

Figure 6-30 Hook up the catheter to a three-way stopcock and flush with heparin.

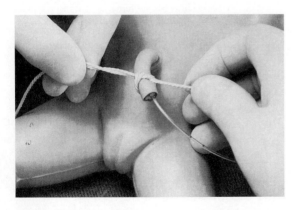

Figure 6-31 Secure the catheter using umbilical tape.

◆ Intraosseous Infusion

Intraosseous (I/O) infusion is defined as a puncture into the medullary cavity of a bone that provides the care provider with a rapid access route for fluids and medications.

Background

The technique of I/O puncture and infusion was first described in the medical literature in 1922. It was used for several decades, but with the development of better intravenous catheters, the procedure lost its popularity until the late 1970s. Even with more advanced catheters, it was still difficult for many skilled physicians to achieve vascular access. Thus there was a reemergence of the procedure, and its acceptance has grown in the prehospital setting.

Generally, I/O infusion is reserved for the pediatric patient up to 6 years of age.

Introduction of a needle into the medullary cavity is relatively rapid and simple, compared to peripheral IV insertion. The procedure only requires the addition of one instrument: a needle with a stylet. There are currently several commercially manufactured I/O or bone marrow biopsy needles available. The needle is usually large bore (12 to 16 gauge), with a shorter shaft than the standard intravenous catheter.

Three sites are suggested for the puncture. The most commonly used site is the proximal tibia, since the tibial plateau has a broad, flat surface. The distal tibia and distal femur can also be accessed.

It should be noted that the I/O IV site is for temporary use only. Once the child's condition has stabilized, another form of intravenous therapy should be initiated. Prolonged use of I/O infusion has proven to lead to infection more often than traditional IVs.

Indications
◆ Cardiac arrest
◆ Multisystem trauma with associated shock and/or severe hypovolemia

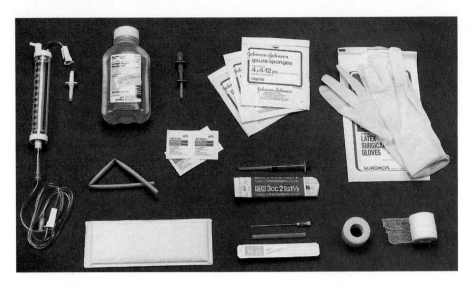

Figure 6-32 Intraosseous infusion equipment.

• Severe dehydration associated with vascular collapse and/or loss of consciousness
• Any child who is unresponsive and in need of immediate drug or fluid resuscitation (burns, status asthmaticus, status epilepticus, sepsis)

Contraindications

• Fracture above the venipuncture site
• Prior infection at the venipuncture site
• Site used for previous venipuncture

Equipment (Figure 6-32)

• Intravenous solution
• IV tubing (microdrip or Buretrol-type)
• Commercial I/O or bone marrow biopsy needle (can substitute large-bore spinal needle)
• Povidone-iodine swabs
• Antibiotic ointment
• 1-inch tape
• Several rolls of 2- or 3-inch Kling
• 10-ml syringe
• Injectable sterile saline
• Pressure pump for volume infusion
• Gloves
• Eye protection (goggles)

Procedure

1. Observe universal precautions.
2. Prepare equipment to be used.
3. Identify the landmark for venipuncture, preferably the anteromedial aspect of the proximal tibia, approximately 1 to 3 cm below the tibial tuberosity (Figure 6-33).
4. Cleanse the puncture site (Figure 6-34).
5. Using a twisting motion, introduce the needle using a 60-degree inferior puncture, away from the joint and epiphyseal plate (Figure 6-35). Note the decrease in resistance as the needle enters the marrow.

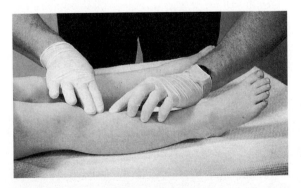

Figure 6-33 The landmark for I/O venipuncture is 1 to 3 cm below the tibial tuberosity.

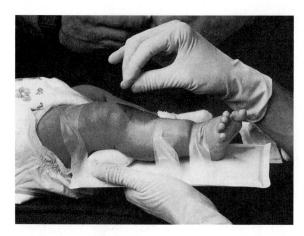

Figure 6-34 Cleanse the puncture site.

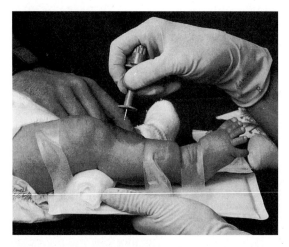

Figure 6-35 Introduce the needle at a 60-degree angle, away from the knee.

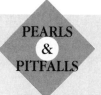

PEARLS
&
PITFALLS

Intraosseous Infusion

I/O infusion is not an elective procedure. It should only be performed when no other vascular access is available. The average patient should be a child in critical condition on whom you have made several unsuccessful IV attempts. However, in special cases, I/O may be the first choice of access.

Complications from I/O infusion have been documented in the medical literature. If the puncture is too shallow, fluid or medication can be infused directly into the tissue, resulting in possible necrosis. If the puncture is too deep, the needle will pierce the opposite side of the bone. Excessive movement of the needle can result in leakage around the bone, thus requiring discontinuance of the IV. Any excessive bleeding following discontinuance will require direct pressure for approximately 10 minutes. Osteomyelitis and fat emboli are complications cited in the literature, but rarely seen.

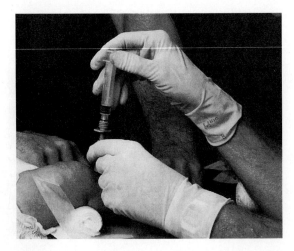

Figure 6-36 Aspirate bone marrow with a 10-cc syringe.

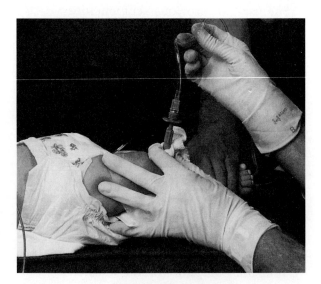

Figure 6-37 Attach the IV line and adjust the flow rate.

6. Remove the stylet.

7. Attach a 10 ml syringe and aspirate bone marrow to verify the location of the needle (Figure 6-36). Remove the syringe.

8. Attach another 10-ml syringe filled with sterile saline. Inject 5 to 10 ml of saline to clear the lumen of the needle.

9. Attach the IV and adjust the flow rate (Figure 6-37).

10. Place antibiotic ointment around the site and secure with tape.

11. Following the administration of a medication, 10 ml of saline should be administered to expedite absorption into the circulatory system.

◆ Pediatric Defibrillation

Defibrillation is the process of sending an electrical current through the myocardial cells to create depolarization. This depolarization allows the heart to initiate a spontaneous organized rhythm.

Background

Pediatric defibrillation differs from the adult method in several ways. First, the pediatric paddle size is much smaller than the adult: 4.5 cm for infants and 8 or 13 cm for older children. Second, the amount of energy delivered to a child is much smaller: 2 J/kg is recommended for initial countershock. In the case of synchronized cardioversion, the procedure is the same as standard defibrillation, except that the synchronizer circuit must be activated by pushing the sync button. A marker will show on the monitor with each QRS complex.

Indications
◆ Ventricular fibrillation
◆ Ventricular tachycardia (pulseless)

Contraindications
◆ A patient with a pulse
◆ Situations in which the act of defibrillating is deemed dangerous, such as a near-drowning patient lying in water near the edge of a swimming pool

Equipment (Figure 6-38)
◆ EKG monitor/defibrillator
◆ Conductive interface (defibrillator gel or pads)

Procedure

1. Establish level of consciousness and evaluate ABCs.

2. Have assistants begin CPR.

3. Turn on EKG monitor/defibrillator, making sure that it is set on PADDLES.

4. Expose the patient's chest and position the patient. (If pediatric paddles are used, position patient supine (Figure 6-39). However,

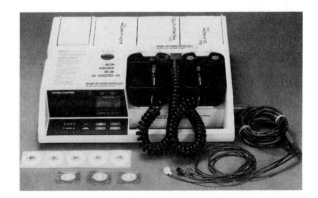

Figure 6-38 Equipment for pediatric defibrillation.

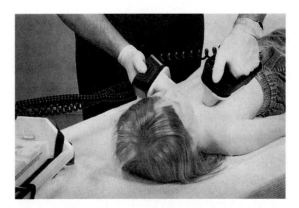

Figure 6-39 Pediatric paddles should be used when available.

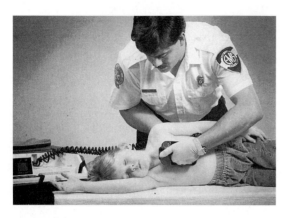

Figure 6-40 Anterior-posterior defibrillation can be performed with adult paddles.

if pediatric paddles are unavailable, adult paddles can be used. Roll the patient into the lateral recumbent position (Figure 6-40).

5. Using interface (gel or pads), perform quick look and verify the need for electrical therapy.

6. Charge the defibrillator to the appropriate joules. The recommendation for pediatric patients is 2 J/kg initially.

7. Reconfirm that the rhythm has not changed and that the pulse is still absent. If the rhythm has changed, reassess the patient and treat accordingly.

8. Call "CLEAR" and visualize the area to verify that no one is in contact with the patient.

9. Apply firm pressure to the paddles and discharge the defibrillator by depressing the two discharge buttons simultaneously.

10. Following countershock, check the patient's pulse and identify the rhythm on the EKG monitor. If the rhythm is unchanged, immediately recharge the defibrillator and countershock at 4 J/kg. If the rhythm changes, treat according to the appropriate American Heart Association algorithm.

◆ Putting It All Together

Any emergency involving a child is always traumatic to all those involved: the child, the family, and the paramedic. Periodic practice in the skills laboratory or emergency department is a good method for retaining those difficult skills, such as IV initiation. Remember that children are not just small adults, and that they do require special attention.

Testing Your Knowledge

1. The smallest diameter of the pediatric airway is located just above the cricoid ring.

   a. True
   b. False

2. The heart rate of a newborn infant is approximately how many beats per minute?

   a. 40 to 60
   b. 60 to 80
   c. 80 to 100
   d. 120 to 160

3. Reflex bradycardia in the infant BEST responds to which of the following drugs?

   a. Atropine sulfate
   b. Oxygen
   c. Dobutamine
   d. Isoproterenol

4. A unique characteristic of the pediatric airway is that the child's:

   a. Larynx is lower (C5-6) than in the adult (C3-4).
   b. Trachea is wider but shorter than in the adult.
   c. Tongue is relatively large compared to the mouth.
   d. Rib cage is rigid with very developed muscles.

5. From the following list of IV sites, select the one that is unique to the pediatric patient under the age of 2 years that can be used by a paramedic.

   a. External jugular vein
   b. Umbilical vein
   c. Scalp vein
   d. Antecubital vein

6. A good rule of thumb to use when selecting an appropriate ETT for a child is:

   a. Use the size that corresponds to the age of the patient.
   b. The ETT should be approximately the same diameter as that of the child's little finger.
   c. Take the weight in kilograms and divide by 3.
   d. The ETT should be approximately the same size as the child's thumb.

7. List two situations when digital intubation is an acceptable option to oral laryngoscopy and intubation.

8. The umbilicus of a newborn has one artery and two veins.

   a. True
   b. False

9. From the following list, select the BEST site for insertion of an intraosseous needle.

   a. Proximal tibial
   b. Distal tibia
   c. Distal femur
   d. Sternum

10. From the following list, select the LEAST appropriate site for starting an IV on a 6-month-old child.

    a. Saphenous vein
    b. Brachial vein
    c. External jugular vein
    d. Scalp vein

Answers are in Appendix A.

BIBLIOGRAPHY

Chameides L, editor: Textbook of Pediatric Advanced Life Support, Dallas, 1988, The American Heart Association and The American Academy of Pediatrics, American Heart Association.

Eichelberger MR, Ball JW, Pratsch GS, et al: *Pediatric emergencies*, ed 1, Englewood Cliffs, NJ, 1992, Brady (Prentice-Hall).

Emergency Medical Technician-Paramedic—National Standard Curriculum: Washington, DC, 1985, US Department of Transportation, US Government Printing Office.

Fleisher G, Ludwig S: *Textbook of pediatric emergency care*, ed 2, Baltimore, 1988, Williams & Wilkens.

Grant H, et al: *Emergency care*, Englewood Cliffs, NJ, 1990, Brady (Prentice-Hall).

Hafen B, Karren K: *Prehospital emergency care and crisis intervention*, ed 3, Englewood, Colo, 1989, Morton Publishing.

Levin DL, et al: *A practical guide to pediatric intensive care*, ed 2, St. Louis, 1984, Mosby.

Manley L, Haley K, Dick M: Intraosseous infusion: rapid vascular access for critically ill or injured infants and children, *J Emerg Nurs* 14(2):63-69, 1988.

Mellick LB, Dierking BH: One size doesn't fit all—choosing pediatric equipment, Part I, *J Emerg Med Serv* 16(6):78-82, 1991.

Mellick LB, Dierking BH: One size doesn't fit all—choosing pediatric equipment, Part II, *J Emerg Med Serv* 16(7):35-46, 1991.

Pediatric Emergencies—EMS Instructor Manual: Washington, DC, 1987, US Department of Health and Human Services and US Department of Transportation, US Government Printing Office.

Pediatric intraosseous infusion training program, Seattle, no date listed, Washington Emergency Medical Services for Children, pp. 1-10.

Simon R, Brenner B: Procedures and techniques in emergency medicine, Baltimore, 1982, Williams & Wilkens.

Smith R et al: Intraosseous infusions by prehospital personnel in critically ill pediatric patients, *Ann Emerg Med* 17(5):491, 1988.

Spivey WH: Intraosseous infusions, *J Pediatr* 111(5)639-643, 1987.

Tsai A, Kallsen G: Epidemiology of pediatric prehospital care, *Ann Emerg Med* 16(3):284, 1987.

Pediatric Endotracheal Intubation

Intubation attempts should not exceed 30 seconds per attempt. If unsuccessful after two attempts, the paramedic should consider alternate airway management techniques. The patient must be hyperventilated between intubation attempts.

Procedure	Possible points	Points awarded
Observe universal precautions.	1	
Assemble laryngoscope blade and handle.	1	
Check light operation.	1	
Check ETT and prepare tape.	1	
Hyperventilate patient.	1	
Insert laryngoscope in right side of mouth and move tongue to left.	1	
Lift upward, avoiding gums or teeth.	1	
Visualize (and verbalize) epiglottis and vocal cords.	1	
Properly insert ETT.	1	
Ventilate patient.	1	
Visualize chest rise.	1	
Check placement of ETT (chest and epigastrium) (one point each).	2	
Secure tube.	1	
Reconfirm tube placement after taping.	1	
TOTAL POINTS	**15**	

COMMENTS _____

_____

_____

Pediatric Digital Intubation

Digital intubation should be utilized if laryngoscopy and oral intubation fails or if the patient has a suspected neck injury. Intubation attempts should not exceed 30 seconds per attempt. If unsuccessful after two attempts, the paramedic should consider alternate airway management techniques. The patient should be hyperventilated between attempts.

Procedure	Possible points	Points awarded
Check ETT and prepare tape.	1	
Hyperventilate patient before intubation attempt.	1	
Position self properly.	1	
Insert middle finger into oropharynx and identify epiglottis.	1	
Introduce ETT properly.	1	
Gently advance tube through glottic opening into trachea.	1	
Remove finger, hold tube, and ventilate the patient.	3	
Confirm tube placement by visualization and auscultation.	2	
Secure tube properly and reassess tube position.	2	
TOTAL POINTS	**13**	

COMMENTS _____

_____

_____

Anterior Pediatric Defibrillation Using Pediatric Paddles

Pediatric paddles are adapters that attach to adult defibrillator paddles. These adapters decrease the surface area that contacts the child's skin. The patient is positioned supine, and the procedure accomplished using the same landmarks as in the adult.

Procedure	Possible points	Points awarded
Ensure adequate CPR.	1	
Prepare equipment.	1	
Bare chest.	1	
Use interface (gel or pads).	1	
Perform quick-look using correct position.	1	
Verify need for electrical therapy.	1	
Charge defibrillator to appropriate level.	1	
Reconfirm rhythm and pulselessness before defibrillation.	2	
Verbally call "clear" and visually clear area.	2	
Apply firm pressure to each paddle.	1	
Deliver countershock.	1	
Check pulse.	1	
Observe and identify rhythm after shock.	1	
Provide appropriate postresuscitation therapy.	2	
Ensure no interruption of CPR >30 seconds.	1	
TOTAL POINTS	**18**	

COMMENTS _____

_____

_____

Anterior/Posterior Pediatric Defibrillation Using Adult Paddles

Defibrillation with adult paddles is accomplished by placing the "sternum" paddle on the anterior surface and the "apex" paddle on the posterior surface of the child. This allows the electrical current to pass directly through the heart muscle.

Procedure	Possible points	Points awarded
Ensure adequate CPR.	1	
Prepare equipment.	1	
Bare chest and roll patient to the side.	1	
Use interface (gel or pads).	1	
Perform quick-look using correct position.	1	
Verify need for electrical therapy.	1	
Charge defibrillator to appropriate level.	1	
Reconfirm rhythm and pulseness before defibrillation.	2	
Verbally call "clear" and visually clear area.	2	
Apply firm pressure to each paddle.	1	
Deliver countershock.	1	
Check pulse.	1	
Observe and identify rhythm after shock.	1	
Provide appropriate postresuscitation therapy.	2	
Ensure no interruption of CPR >30 seconds	1	
TOTAL POINTS	**18**	

COMMENTS _____

_____

_____

Cannulation of Peripheral Veins of the Upper or Lower Extremity

The vessels of the arms and legs are commonly used for intravenous initiation in most children. Intravenous sites must be selected carefully, since most pediatric veins are very fragile and readily collapse.

Procedure	Possible points	Points awarded
Observe universal precautions.	1	
Assemble necessary equipment.	1	
Select and prepare solution (includes connecting and flushing tubing; checking for expiration, clarity, and leaks).	4	
Restrain patient.	1	
Place tourniquet proximal to the IV site.	1	
Locate suitable vein and cleanse site.	1	
Correctly perform venipuncture using over-the-needle catheter. Note blood return.	2	
Advance catheter and remove needle.	1	
Release tourniquet.	1	
Attach IV tubing and slowly introduce fluid into vein.	1	
Adjust flow rate.	1	
Secure catheter.	1	
Reconfirm flow rate and check for IV patency.	1	
TOTAL POINTS	**17**	

COMMENTS _____

_____

_____

Cannulation of Peripheral Scalp Veins

The scalp veins are rarely used in critical situations because they are small, fragile, and often difficult to access. They are useful in administering fluids and medications when other intravenous sites are unavailable as a result of poor vascular status or trauma.

Procedure	Possible points	Points awarded
Observe universal precautions.	1	
Assemble necessary equipment.	1	
Select and prepare solution (includes connecting and flushing tubing; checking for expiration, clarity, and leaks).	4	
Restrain patient.	1	
Place rubberband tournquet around superior aspect of head.	1	
Locate suitable vein and prepare skin (may require shaving).	1	
Flush butterfly needle or over-the-needle catheter with sterile solution.	1	
Stretch skin over vein and identify blood flow direction.	1	
Cleanse venipuncture site.	1	
Correctly perform venipuncture and note blood return.	2	
Advance needle or catheter.	1	
Release tourniquet.	1	
Attach IV tubing and slowly introduce fluid into vein.	1	
Adjust flow rate.	1	
Secure needle or catheter.	1	
Reconfirm flow rate and check for IV patency.	1	
TOTAL POINTS	**20**	

COMMENTS

Intraosseous Cannulation

I/O infusion allows for the administration of fluids and drugs via the intramedullary cavity into the circulatory system. It must be realized that this procedure is to be used in life or death situations after a minimum of two peripheral intravenous attempts have proven unsuccessful.

Procedure	Possible points	Points awarded
Assemble equipment.	1	
Identify landmark for puncture.	1	
Cleanse puncture site.	1	
Use appropriate needle and correctly perform puncture into intramedullary cavity. Insert at a 60 degree angle, using firm pressure and rotary motion.	1	
Remove stylet.	1	
Attach 10-ml syringe (filled with 5 ml of saline) and aspirate bone marrow to verify placement.	1	
Inject 3 to 4 ml of saline to clear lumen of needle.	1	
Attach IV line and regulate flow rate.	2	
Place antibiotic ointment around site and secure with padding and tape.	1	
TOTAL POINTS	**10**	

COMMENTS _____

_____

_____

Umbilical Vein Catheterization

Umbilical vein catheterization is used in the neonate when rapid IV access is required. The umbilicus has one large artery and two small veins which can be accessed. In the prehospital setting, the vein is recommended for catheterization.

Procedure	Possible points	Points awarded
Prepare necessary equipment.	1	
Restrain infant.	1	
Cleanse and drape area. Cleanse umbilicus with povidone-iodine solution.	1	
Identify umbilical veins.	1	
Dilate lumen of vein with hemostat.	1	
Introduce and advance the umbilical catheter until blood return is noted.	1	
Hook catheter to three-way stopcock and flush with 1 ml of heparin.	2	
Secure catheter using umbilical tape.	1	
Hook up IV tubing.	1	
Monitor for bleeding.	1	
TOTAL POINTS	**11**	

COMMENTS _____

_____

_____

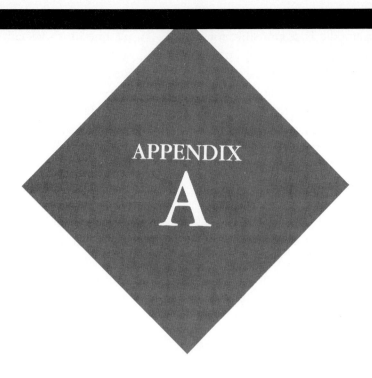

APPENDIX

A

Answer Key

◆ Chapter 1: Patient Evaluation

1. a   Evaluation of the scene
   b   Identification of life-threatening illness or injury
   c   Rapid intervention
   d   Comprehensive assessment
   e   Treatment and transportation
   f   Reevaluation
2. a   Establishing the responsiveness of a patient is typically the first thing accomplished by a paramedic. This can be done by speaking to the conscious patient or stimulating the unresponsive patient.
3. d   A thorough paramedic should obtain information from all available sources, including the patient, first responders, and family members.
4. c   The goal of the primary survey is to identify life-threatening emergencies.
5. A, Evaluate and establish an *airway*.

B, Evaluate and establish *breathing*.
C, Evaluate *circulation*, control bleeding, and begin CPR if necessary.
D, *Disability* is a mini-neurologic examination, based on alertness, verbal and painful response, and determination of unresponsiveness.
E, *Expose* the patient completely to perform an assessment and locate injuries.

6. Airway patency is the ability to move air into and out of the lungs for the purpose of gas exchange.
7. b   Questions such as "Was the fire arson or accidentally set?" are not appropriate. This type of question provides you with no information that will affect the patient's care or outcome.
8. d   The chief complaint is often described as being the answer to the question "Why did you call for the ambulance today?" It is the direct quote stating the patient's main ailment.

9. d   The paramedic is responsible for thoroughly evaluating the patient and providing competent medical care and transportation to a medical facility.

10. b   Nausea, headache, and thirst, are all subjective information, since these are symptoms that only the patient can confirm.

11. a   Both the anterior and posterior surface of the body must be examined in the primary survey. This assures the paramedic that no life-threatening injuries such as open thoracic wounds escape recognition and treatment.

12. a   In the case of critical patients requiring advanced airway and circulatory management, the paramedic may never exit the primary resuscitation phase.

13. A, Alert
    V, Verbal response
    P, Painful response
    U, Unresponsive

14. A, Allergies
    M, Medications
    P, Pertinent past medical history
    L, Last oral intake
    E, Events leading up to the emergency

◆ Chapter 2: Advanced Airway Management

1. b   The epiglottis is a cartilaginous fold that prevents aspiration of food, water and saliva into the trachea.

2. The three axes of alignment necessary for proper intubation: the oropharyngeal, the pharyngoglottic, and the glototracheal axes.

3. a   When suctioning a patient orally, the paramedic should suction no longer than **10** seconds. Similarly, tracheal suctioning should last no longer than **5** seconds.

4. d   Direct laryngoscopy allows the paramedic to visualize the upper airway, allowing him to intubate or remove foreign bodies using Magill forceps.

5. a   Endotracheal intubation should take no longer than 30 seconds. If you exceed this time period, the patient should be hyperventilated and intubation reattempted.

6. d   Patient "a" is semi-responsive and may still have a gag reflex, patient "b" has possible esophageal varices secondary to alcohol abuse (possible hemorrhage), and patient "c" is too young for consideration (16 years-old is the minimum age limit for EOA insertion).

7. b   False. In addition, the EGTA tube does not have holes near the proximal end of the tube. Ventilation is accomplished via a separate hole in the mask.

8. a   True. The PTL and ETC are designed for placement in either the trachea or esophagus, with the operator then ventilating in the appropriate tube.

9. c   From the given list, all are considered muscle relaxants except for haloperidol, which is considered a major tranquilizer.

10. The are five major contraindications for performing nasotracheal intubation:
    Apnea
    Airway obstruction
    Severe facial injury
    Basilar skull fracture
    Bleeding disorders

11. a   True. Cricothyrotomy is used as a last effort to obtain an airway, when other methods have failed. The procedure may result in many complications.

12. c   Percutaneous transtracheal ventilation is also known as needle cricothyrotomy.

◆ Chapter 3: Circulatory Management

1. Trouser, diaper, logroll
2. c   The intercostal spaces widen due to increased intrathoracic pressure
3. a   True—Blood vessels and nerves supplying the chest wall are located on the underside of each rib.
4. c   Congestive heart failure would likely include pulmonary edema; thus PASG application would increase respiratory distress.
5. d   Tension pneumothorax would result in hyperresonance over the affected side due to trapped air in the pleural cavity.
6. c   A simple pneumothorax will often result following an incorrect puncture.
7. d   One would see a progressively decreasing drip rate with IV infiltration.
8. d   The largest bore possible should always be initiated in the adult shock patient, preferably 14 gauge.
9. d   A catheter embolus is a potential complication from reinsertion of a needle through a plastic catheter.
10. d   Answers a and b are correct. One should never tap on the neck of a patient; this action could possibly stimulate the patient vagally or even create an embolus if the patient suffers from atherosclerotic neck vessels.
11. a   True—This patient is in need of an IV lifeline, both for giving immediate medications such as furosemide and morphine, as well as other medications, should her condition deteriorate.
12. a   True—The external jugular vein is a peripheral IV site and is used by many EMS systems as a back-up site should the arms not provide venous access.

◆ Chapter 4: Medication Administration

1. b   The subcutaneous layer of tissue is also called the "fatty" layer.
2. c   Epinephrine 1:1,000 is given most often by paramedics subcutaneously for allergic and asthmatic episodes.
3. a   True—Poor perfusion can seriously alter absorption rates of medications.
4. b   False—Intravenous and endotracheal administration of a medication provides the most rapid routes of absorption.
5. d   Intramuscular injections are given at a 90-degree angle.
6. a   Intravenous bolus (IV push) is the most commonly used route of drug administration used in the prehospital setting.
7. a   True—Intravenous drip is used for titration or continuous medication administration.
8. N, Narcan (or naloxone)
   A, atropine
   V, Valium
   E, epinephrine
   L, lidocaine
9. a   True—All patients receiving ET bolus medications should be provided with hyperventilation before and after administration.
10. a   True—Because of the side effects of most bronchodilators, continuous EKG monitoring is recommended.

◆ Chapter 5: Cardiac Skills

1. b   Lead II provides the best electrical picture because its position is very near the normal electrical axis of the heart.

2. a   True. Although the quick-look paddles allow for rapid EKG interpretation and defibrillation, they do not provide for effective long-term cardiac monitoring of the patient.

3. d   The cardioscope does not function with a heat stylus; only the recorder uses a heat stylus.

4. d   a and c are the correct answers. Defibrillation and unsynchronized cardioversion are considered to be the same procedure.

5. b   False—Children can either be countershocked using pediatric paddles, or by using adult paddles which are placed on the patient's chest and back (between the scapulae).

6. c   A 44-lb child weighs 20 kg (1 lb = 2.2 kg). Initial pediatric defibrillation is performed, using the formula of 2 joules/kg: (20 kg × 2 joules/kg = 40 joules).

7. c   Synchronized cardioversion monitors the EKG for the R-wave. By discharging on this wave, it avoids the relative refractory period and prevents the onset of ventricular fibrillation or ventricular tachycardia.

8. The two most commonly used forms of vagal maneuver used in the prehospital setting are Valsalva's maneuver and carotid sinus massage.

9. a   True—CVA, bradycardia, or asystole can be seen following a vagal maneuver, the latter two resulting from increased vagal tone.

10. a   External pacing is not indicated in ventricular fibrillation.

11. b   False. Electrical capture of a noninvasive cardiac pacemaker is usually represented on an EKG by a wide QRS complex and a tall, broad T-wave.

◆ Chapter 6: Advanced Pediatric Skills

1. b   The smallest diameter of the pediatric airway is subglottic, just inferior to the cricoid ring.

2. d   The average heart rate for a newborn infant ranges from 120 to 160 beats per minute.

3. b   Reflex bradycardia is very responsive to oxygen in the pediatric patient.

4. c   Proportionately, the child's tongue is relatively large compared to the mouth.

5. c   Scalp veins provide an alternate IV site in very young children and may be used as an optional site if necessary.

6. b   The diameter of the child's little finger provides the paramedic a quick reference when selecting an endotracheal tube for the pediatric patient.

7. a.   When the paramedic is unable to successfully intubate the patient by laryngoscopy.
   b.   If cervical neck injury is suspected.

8. a   The umbilicus of a newborn has one artery and two veins. This is an excellent site for emergency venous access and is a relatively simple procedure to perform.

9. a   The best site for an intraosseous infusion is located 1 to 3 cm distal to the tibial tuberosity on the anteromedial surface of the lower leg.

10. c   The external jugular vein on young children is very difficult to locate and cannulate. The average 6-month-old has a very short, stocky neck, which does not provide for proper landmark identification.

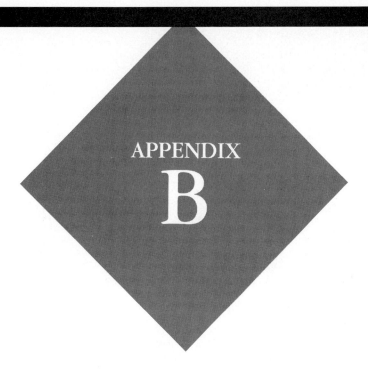

APPENDIX B

Nasogastric Tube Insertion

Objectives

A paramedic should be able to—

1. Discuss nasogastric (NG) tube insertion both from an anatomic and a procedural standpoint.

2. List three indications for NG tube insertion.

3. List one contraindication to NG tube insertion.

4. Given an adult intubation manneqin, demonstrate the procedure for insertion of NG tube.

Insertion of an NG tube is the placement of a specialized suction catheter through the nose, down the esophagus, and into the stomach to remove stomach contents.

Indications

NG tube insertion is indicated when evacuation of stomach contents such as air or food is required. An NG tube may also be inserted to dilute or lavage ingested poisons or to remove blood when the patient has gastrointestinal hemorrhage.

Contraindications

An NG tube should not be inserted through the nose of a patient with severe facial trauma. The patient may have a fracture of the cribriform plate, resulting in accidental placement of the tube into the cranial cavity. The tube may be inserted orally at the direction of Medical Control. In addition, NG tubes should not be inserted in a patient with possible epiglottitis or croup.

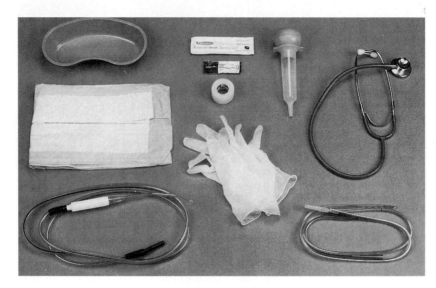

Figure B-1 Equipment for NG tube insertion.

Things to Remember...

The NG tube may have been affected by the temperature in the emergency vehicle. If the tube is too soft and pliable, place it in an emesis basin of ice for a few minutes. If cold and stiff, insert it in an emesis basin full of warm water.

A common error is to insert the tip of the tube upward, which causes the tube to get caught in the turbinates, causing the patient pain and bleeding.

The tube may inadvertently pass into the trachea. If this happens the patient will begin to cough and choke. Pull the tube back into the posterior pharynx and advance it again. Placing the patient in a sitting position with the head slightly flexed on the chest may avoid this problem.

If you are unable to insert the tube to the predetermined measurement, the tube is probably in the patient's trachea or curled in the mouth or throat. Look in the mouth, then withdraw the tube slightly.

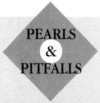

PEARLS & PITFALLS

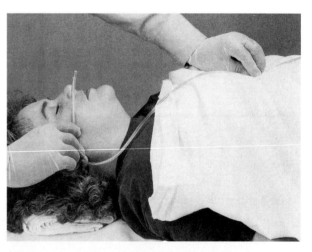

Figure B-2 Measure the tube from the patient's earlobe to the tip of the nose, then to the bottom of the xiphoid process.

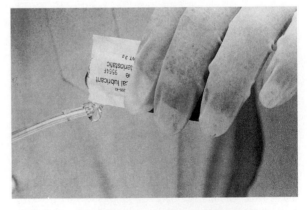

Figure B-3 Lubricate the tube with water-soluble gel.

Equipment (Figure B-1)

- NG tube
- 50-ml irrigation syringe
- Water-soluble lubricant
- Adhesive tape
- Saline for irrigation
- Emesis basin
- Gloves

Procedure

1. Assess the need for NG tube insertion.
2. Use universal precautions.
3. Assemble the needed equipment.
4. Explain the procedure to the patient.
5. If possible, have the patient sitting up. Use a pad or towel to protect the patient's clothing.
6. Give the patient a handful of tissues because this procedure may cause tearing. An emesis basin should also be handy in case the patient vomits as a result of stimulation of the gag reflex.
7. Look at the nose for deformity or obstruction that may make it difficult to insert an NG tube. Determine the best side for insertion, usually the patient's right nostril.
8. Measure the tube from the patient's earlobe to the tip of the nose. Then measure from the earlobe to the bottom of the xiphoid process. Total these two measurements and mark the correct length on the tube with adhesive tape (Figure B-2).
9. Lubricate 6 to 8 inches of the tube with water-soluble gel (Figure B-3).
10. Insert the tube in one of the nostrils and gently advance it toward the posterior nasopharynx. It is easiest if you direct the tube toward the patient's ear (Figure B-4).
11. When you feel the tube at the nasopharyngeal junction, rotate it 180 degrees inward toward the other nostril. Gently advance the tube until it is in the nasopharynx.
12. As the tube enters the oropharynx, instruct the patient to swallow.
13. Pass the tube to the predetermined point. (Do not force the tube if resistance is encountered.)
14. Check the placement of the tube by two methods: aspirate gastric contents; and place a stethoscope over the epigastric region and auscultate while injecting 20 to 30 ml of air into the tube (Figure B-5).

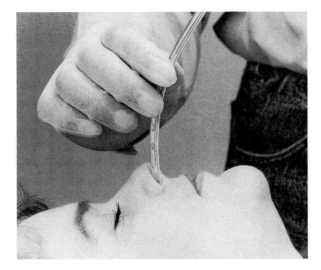

Figure B-4 Insert the tube into the nose and advance it directly toward the posterior nasopharynx.

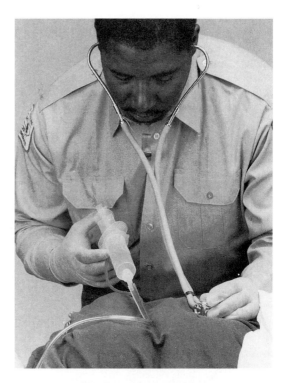

Figure B-5 Check the placement of the NG tube.

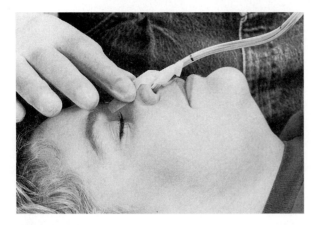

Figure B-6 Tape tube in place; connect to low suction, if ordered.

15. Tape the tube in place and connect to low suction, if ordered (Figure B-6).

16. Document the procedure, including the following information: size of tube inserted, degree of difficulty, tube placement checked, complications such as bleeding or vomiting, and name of person performing the procedure (Figure B-7).

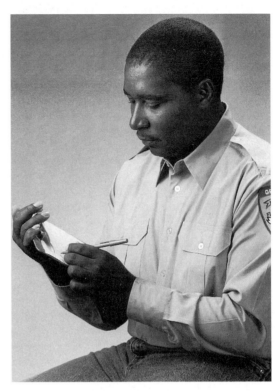

Figure B-7 Provide thorough documentation.

BIBLIOGRAPHY

Budassi S, Barber J: *Mosby's manual of emergency care: practice and procedures,* ed 2, St. Louis, 1984, Mosby.

California Emergency Care: Student handbook EMT-P skills test, ed 4, Lafayette, Calif, 1983, California Emergency Care Standards and Training.

Caroline N: *Emergency care in the streets,* ed 3, Boston, 1987, Little, Brown.

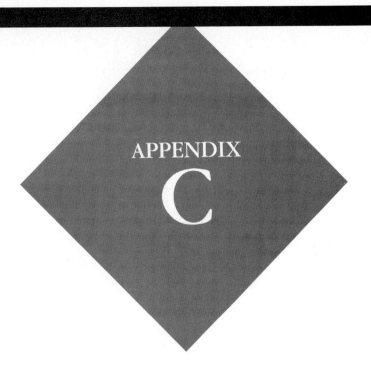

Urinary Catheter Insertion

Objectives

A paramedic should be able to—

1. Describe urinary catheter insertion.

2. List two indications for urinary catheter insertion.

3. List two contraindications to urinary catheter insertion.

4. Using a catheterization mannequin, demonstrate the procedure for insertion of a urinary catheter in both the male and female patient.

U rinary catheter insertion is placement of a drainage tube through the meatus into the urinary bladder to drain urine.

Indications

Catheterization is indicated for drainage of the urinary bladder to precisely measure urine output, or when there is loss of bladder control. In the acute setting, it is more commonly used when the patient who is in congestive heart failure has been given a potent diuretic, such as furosemide.

Contraindications

Urinary catheterization has relatively few contraindications in the prehospital setting. Blood at the meatus of a trauma patient or past history of urethral stricture are two of the most common.

Equipment (Figure C-1)

- Disposable sterile bladder catheter kit
- Water-soluble lubricating jelly
- Plastic-coated drape
- Drape with pre-cut opening

◆ Cleansing solution
◆ Sterile gloves
◆ Prefilled syringe containing sterile water
◆ Correct size urinary catheter
◆ Clamp
◆ Connecting tubing and collecting bag

Procedure

Female patients

1. Assess the need for catheter insertion.

2. Assemble the needed equipment.

3. Explain the procedure to the patient.

4. Use universal precautions.

5. Lay patient flat on her back, if possible, with hips bent and abducted. Place her feet approximately 24 inches apart. Make sure you have good lighting.

6. Place the sterile catheter kit between her legs and open kit aseptically. Open the Foley catheter and drop the catheter into the open kit, taking care not to contaminate the catheter.

7. Put on the sterile gloves. Test the balloon on the Foley catheter by injecting it with sterile water from the prefilled syringe.

8. Ask the patient to raise her pelvis by pushing down with her feet. Insert drape under her buttocks. Instruct patient to lower her pelvis onto the drape (Figure C-2).

9. Position the pre-cut drape so the opening is over the patient's perineal area (Figure C-3).

10. Open the packet of lubricating jelly and

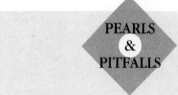

Aseptic Technique

Aseptic technique is of great importance and must be emphasized. Unsterile conditions may result in unnecessary infection, urosepsis, and possibly death. Good technique is a must!

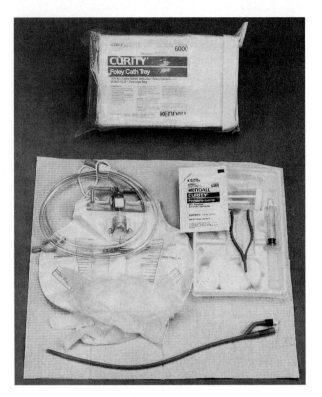

Figure C-1   Equipment for urinary catheter insertion.

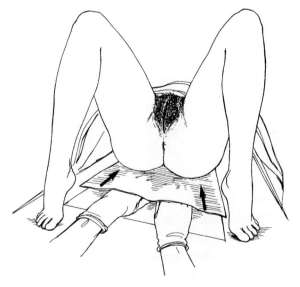

Figure C-2   Place a drape under the patient's buttocks.

squeeze a small amount onto a sterile gauze pad or into one of the container dividers.

11. Open the cleansing solution and pour the solution over the cotton balls.

12. If you are right handed, use your gloved left hand to spread the patient's labia so the meatus is exposed. REMEMBER: Your left hand is now considered contaminated (Figure C-4).

13. Pick up the forceps with your right hand. Pick up the solution-soaked cotton balls one by one. Wipe one time in a downward motion to cleanse the urethral meatus. Discard the cotton ball. Repeat the procedure, using the remaining cotton balls (Figure C-5).

14. Using your uncontaminated hand, pick up the catheter and gently insert it 2 to 3 inches into the urethral opening. Be gentle and never force the catheter. If you break sterile technique at any point you must start over with a new sterile kit (Figure C-6).

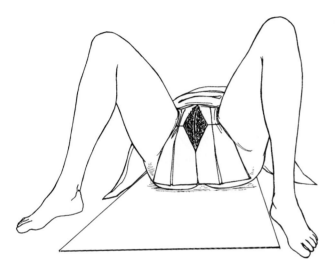

Figure C-3 Place the pre-cut drape over the perineal area.

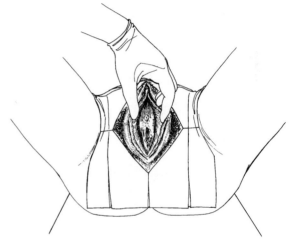

Figure C-4 Expose the meatus by spreading the patient's labia.

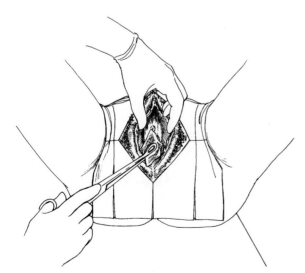

Figure C-5 Cleanse the urethral meatus.

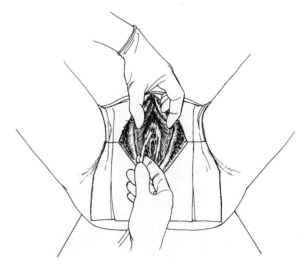

Figure C-6 Insert the catheter into the urethral opening using sterile technique.

15. As the catheter enters the bladder, urine will return. Advance the catheter an additional 2 to 3 inches past the point where urine return was obtained. (This will avoid urethral damage when the balloon is inflated.) Release the labia.

16. Attach the prefilled syringe to the Y portion of the catheter and instill the sterile water. The correct amount required for each catheter is written on the catheter.

17. Connect the open end of the catheter to the drainage tube and collection bag. This step can be done when you first open the kit.

18. If more than 1000 ml drains into the bag, clamp the tube and notify Medical Control.

19. Tape the drainage tube to the patient's inner thigh.

20. Document the size of catheter, ease of insertion, amount and color of urine obtained, complications, date, and time.

Male patients

1. Assess the need for catheter insertion.

2. Assemble the needed equipment.

3. Explain the procedure to the patient.

4. Use universal precautions.

5. Position patient flat on his back, if possible. Place the plastic-coated drape across the patient's thighs.

6. Pull the penis through the opening of the pre-cut drape (Figure C-7). Whichever hand you used is now considered contaminated.

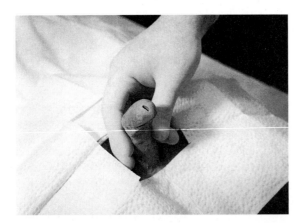

Figure C-7 Pull the penis through the opening in the pre-cut drape.

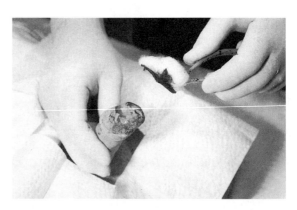

Figure C-8 Cleanse the area.

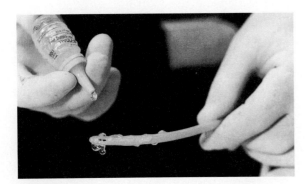

Figure C-9 Lubricate the first 7 to 10 inches of the catheter.

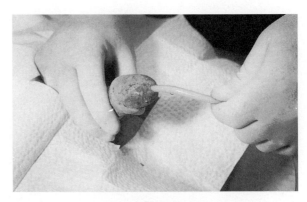

Figure C-10 Advance the catheter 7 to 10 inches.

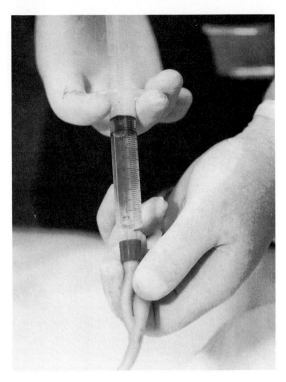

Figure C-11   Attach a syringe filled with water to the Y portion of the catheter.

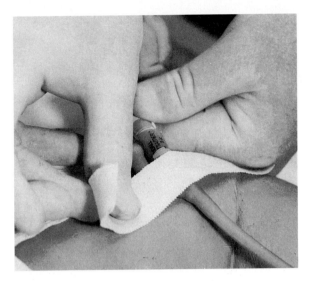

Figure C-12   Tape the drainage tube to the patient's inner thigh or the abdomen.

7. Hold the shaft of the penis perpendicular to his body while you cleanse the area (Figure C-8).

8. If he is not circumcised, remember to pull back the foreskin before cleansing and insertion. (After catheter insertion, remember to pull the foreskin forward again.)

9. Lubricate the first 7 to 10 inches of the catheter, since the male urethra is longer (Figure C-9).

10. Using your sterile hand, advance the catheter 7 to 10 inches. If you feel some resistance where the prostate gland is located, decrease the angle of the penis (Figure C-10).

11. Once urine begins to flow, advance the catheter another 2 to 3 inches.

12. Attach the prefilled syringe to the Y portion of the catheter and instill the sterile water (Figure C-11). The correct amount required for each catheter is written on the catheter.

13. Connect the open end of the catheter to the drainage tube and collection bag. This step can be done when you first open the kit.

14. If more than 1000 ml drains into the bag, clamp the tube, and notify Medical Control.

15. Tape the drainage tube to the patient's inner thigh or the abdomen (Figure C-12).

16. Document the size of catheter, ease of insertion, amount and color of urine obtained, complications, date, and time.

BIBLIOGRAPHY

Budassi S, Barber J: *Mosby's manual of emergency care: practice and procedures*, ed 2, St. Louis, 1984, Mosby.

Caroline N: *Emergency care in the streets*, ed 3, Boston, 1987, Little, Brown.

California Emergency Care: Student handbook EMT—P skills test, ed 4, Lafayette, Calif, 1983, California Emergency Care Standards and Training.

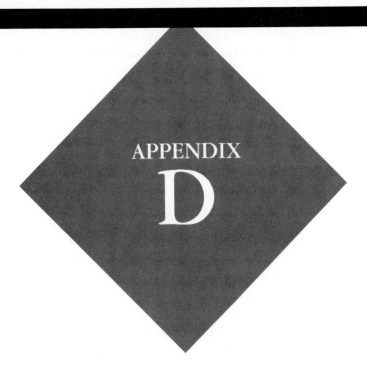

Thrombolytic Therapy in the Prehospital Setting

Objectives

A paramedic should be able to—

1. State the definition of thrombolysis.

2. State the primary indication for thrombolytic therapy in the prehospital setting.

3. List three thrombolytic agents used for myocardial infarction.

Thrombolysis is the breaking up of a thrombus, or blood clot, that obstructs a blood vessel.

Intravenous thrombolytic therapy improves left ventricular function and reduces mortality in patients with acute myocardial infarction. The effectiveness of thrombolytic therapy for myocardial infarction is inversely related to the time interval before it is given. Therefore, administration of thrombolytic agents by prehospital care providers has been proposed to shorten time between the onset of myocardial infarction and definitive therapy.

As of 1993, prehospital administration of thrombolytic agents for myocardial infarction should still be considered experimental. In European and Middle Eastern trials, prehospital delivery of thrombolytic agents by physician-directed mobile intensive care units has been successful in aborting infarcts (Dalzell, Purvis, Adgey; Gibler, Kereiakes, Dean, et al). Clinical trials in the United States have shown that few patients evaluated in the prehospital setting are actual candidates for thrombolytic therapy. Combining projects from Nashville and Cincinnati, only 27 of 562 total patients with chest pain (4.8%) were candidates for prehospital thrombolysis. In addition, a decline in paramedic skills has been noted because of the infrequent administration of thrombolytics. The authors of these studies concluded that "substantial allocation of financial and human resources for prehospital delivery of intravenous thrombolytic therapy does not appear warranted" (Gibler, Kereiakes, Dean, et al).

Another study has pointed out that prehospital approaches to thrombolytic therapy have the potential to shorten the time to thrombolytic therapy in only a minority of the affected U.S. population because only approximately half of acute myocardial infarction patients are transported by the EMS system. Other potential problems include the high cost of electrocardiographic and communication equipment by ambulance, field drugs, cost and breakage, and additional medicolegal risks for physicians and prehospital care providers (Ornato, 1990).

A prehospital approach that may reduce the time from onset of myocardial infarction to thrombolytic therapy has been to transmit the 12-lead EKG signal directly from the field to the hospital. In a study by Karagounis et al, an infield EKG caused negligible delays in paramedic time and led to significant decreases in time to in-hospital thrombolytic therapy (Karagounis, Ipsen, Jessop). In another study the time from admission to the hospital to initiation of thrombolytic therapy was determined to be 83 ± 55 minutes. Shorter hospital time delays were observed in patients in whom a prehospital EKG was obtained as part of a protocol-driven prehospital diagnostic strategy and a diagnosis of acute infarction made before arrival at the hospital (36.3 ± 11.3 minutes). These authors concluded that the "implementation of a protocol-driven prehospital diagnostic strategy may be associated with a reduction in time to thrombolytic therapy" (Kereiakes, Weaver, Anderson, et al, 1990).

In summary, although thrombolytic therapy for acute myocardial infarction in the field is experimental, data seem to indicate that there are only a few patients who would actually benefit from prehospital thrombolytic therapy, and that there are many logistic, cost, and medicolegal factors that may be prohibitive. However, transmitting the EKG from the field to the hospital to assist with more rapid diagnosis of myocardial infarction may be practical, as well as extremely important in reducing the time to thrombolytic therapy.

The following indications, contraindications, and procedures* are rapidly changing. The Medical Director of your system should be contacted for your system's current status referable to thrombolytic therapy.

Indications

- Chest discomfort typical for myocardial ischemia that lasts at least 30 minutes and is unresponsive to sublingual nitroglycerin
- Discomfort generally less than 6 hours' duration
- EKG evidence of myocardial infarction as determined by Medical Control from his/her review of the EKG transmitted from the field to the hospital

Contraindications
Absolute
- Active internal bleeding
- History of cerebral vascular accident in previous 2 months
- Known intracranial neoplasm (tumor), arteriovenous malformation, or aneurysm
- History of intracranial surgery or trauma, intraspinal surgery or trauma within previous 2 months
- Hemorrhagic retinopathy such as proliferative retinopathy
- Uncontrolled, severe hypertension ($\geq 200/120$ mm Hg)

*Adapted from a document by the Cardiology Section of the Department of Medicine, East Carolina University School of Medicine, March, 1991.

- Previous significant allergic reaction to antistreplase or streptokinase
- Recent surgery or trauma ($<$2 weeks) that could be a source for bleeding
- Inability to rule out aortic dissection
- Prolonged or traumatic cardiopulmonary resuscitation

Relative
- Recent surgery or trauma ($\geq$2 weeks)
- Active peptic ulcer disease
- Severe liver disease or renal disease
- Current use of anticoagulants/preexisting bleeding disorder
- Women of childbearing potential/pregnancy

Table D-1   Individual Agents

Streptokinase/Streptase	rt-PA/Activase	Antistreplase/Eminase
Pharmacology		
Streptokinase forms an "activator complex" with plasminogen and converts plasminogen to plasmin. Plasmin subsequently degrades fibrin clots as well as other plasma proteins, including fibrinogen.	rt-PA—a serine protease that converts plasminogen to plasmin after binding to fibrin in a thrombus and thus initiating "local fibrinolysis."	Antistreplase—a synthetic derivative of streptokinase-plasminogen complex with the active center of the complex temporarily blocked by an anisoyl group. The active complex converts plasminogen to plasmin in thrombi and in blood.
Reconstitution		
To the 1,500,000 U bottle add slowly 5 ml of NS to D_5W for injection, USP, directing it at the side of the vial. Roll and tilt to reconstitute. Avoid shaking, because it may cause foaming. Add an additional 40 ml of diluent to the vial, avoiding agitation. Then administer via infusion pump.	Reconstitute aseptically by adding 50 ml of sterile H_2O for injection, USP, to 50-mg vial. Direct diluent to side of vial to avoid excessive foaming. Use rt-PA as soon as possible after reconstitution, since it contains no antibacterial preservatives. Inspect for particulate matter and then administer via separate IV line as below.	Reconstitute only with 5 ml of sterile H_2O for injection, USP. Direct diluent against side of vial. Gently roll. Do not shake. Avoid foaming. Inspect for particulate material. Withdraw entire contents of vial 30 U; do not dilute further before administration. Must use within 30 minutes of reconstitution.
Thrombolytic therapy		
After pretreating with Benadryl, 50 mg, intravenously and methylprednisolone (Solu-Medrol), 100 mg, intravenously or equivalent steroid: Begin 1,500,000 IU streptokinase intravenously over 60 minutes via separate IV line After 4 hours, give 5000 U of heparin bolus intravenously followed by continuous infusion at 1000 U/hour.	Begin heparin and rt-PA simultaneously. Give heparin, 5000 U bolus, intravenously and continuous infusion at 1000 U/hour. Give rt-PA, 10 mg bolus, over 2 minutes, followed by 50 mg intravenously over first hour; then 20 mg/hour for 2 hr, for a total dosage of 100 mg.	After pretreating with Benadryl, 50 mg, intravenously and methylprednisolone, 100 mg, intravenously or equivalent steroid: Inject the entire 30 U of antistreplase intravenously over 2 to 5 minutes. After injection, flush IV line with D_5W or ½ NS. 4 to 6 hours after antistreplase, give bolus of 5000 U heparin and follow with continuous infusion at 1000 U/hour.

PEARLS
&
PITFALLS

Thrombolytic Therapy

1. Initiate treatment as soon as directed by medical control.
2. Minimize arterial and venous punctures. (Hold pressure for at least 30 min.)
3. Avoid noncompressible vessel punctures (e.g., internal jugular).
4. If serious bleeding occurs, discontinue thrombolytic therapy, hold heparin.
5. Monitor for signs/symptoms of bleeding:
   a. Assess all existing hematomas/ venipuncture sites.
   b. Change in mental status or neurologic examination may signal intracranial hemorrhage.
   c. New back/leg pain may indicate retroperitoneal bleeding.
6. Avoid Foley catheters.
7. Monitor for allergic reactions and treat by discontinuing thrombolytic agent, parenteral antihistamines, steroids, and pressors, as indicated.
8. Be alert to appearance of certain dysrhythmias and their treatment:
   a. Ventricular ectopy: lidocaine infusion
   b. Symptomatic bradycardia: atropine, isoproterenol, pacemaker
   c. Accelerated idioventricular rhythm: observation
9. Avoid excessive movement and unintentional physical trauma to patients (lifting, pushing, tugging, restraints).
10. Avoid intramuscular injections.
11. Monitor for hypotension, cardiac tamponade, pulmonary edema, and reocclusion.
12. Blood sampling should be through preexisting line with three-way stopcock, if possible.

- Serious advanced illness
- Acute pericarditis/pericardial rub
- Subacute bacterial endocarditis
- Known left heart thrombus
- Prior exposure to any streptokinase-containing agent (antistreplase or streptokinase), especially if within previous 6 months
- Septic thrombophlebitis
- Indwelling nasogastric tube or endotracheal tube
- Recent puncture of noncompressible vessel
- Age >75 years old
- Severe anemia

Procedure

1. Observe universal precautions.

2. Draw blood for the following laboratory studies: CBC, PT/PTT, platelets, fibrinogen, type and screen for packed cells, electrolytes, BUN, creatinine, CPK with isoenzymes.

3. If not allergic, have patient chew 325 mg of buffered aspirin.

4. Start two peripheral intravenous lines in different arms: one for the thrombolytic agent and one for the administration of adjunct parenteral therapy.

5. Have emergency medications available: lidocaine for ventricular dysrhythmias; diphenhydramine for allergic reactions (administer intravenously); solumedrol for allergic reactions; and dopamine, epinephrine, atropine, and nitroglycerin.

6. After selecting the thrombolytic agent of choice, initiate infusion as described in Table D-1.

7. Do not mix any other medication/diluent in the vial containing the thrombolytic agent.

BIBLIOGRAPHY

Dalzell GW, Previs J, Adgey A: The initial electrocardiogram in patients seen by a mobile coronary care unit, *Q J Med* 78(287):227-33, 1991.

Gibler WB, Kereiakes DJ, Dean EN, et al: Prehospital diagnosis and treatment of acute myocardial infarction: a north-south perspective: the Cincinnati Heart Project and the Nashville Prehospital TPA Trial, *Am Heart J* 121(1) (Part 1):1-11, 1991.

Karagounis L, Ipsen SK, Jessop MR, et al: Impact of filed transmitted electrocardiography on time to in-hospital thrombolytic therapy and acute myocardial infarction, *Am J Cardiol* 66(10):786-91, 1990.

Kereiakes DJ, Weaver WD, Anderson JL, et al: Time delays in the diagnosis and treatment of acute myocardial infarction: a tale of eight cities: report from Prehospital Study Group and the Cincinnati Heart Project, *Am Heart J* 120(4)773-80, 1990.

Ornato JP: The earliest thrombolytic treatment of acute myocardial infarction: ambulance or emergency department? *Clin Cardiol* 13(suppl 8):27-31, 1990.

Schoefer J, Butner J, Geng G, et al: Prehospital thrombolysis and acute myocardial infarction, *Am J Cardiol* 66:1429-33, 1990.

Thrombolytic Protocol from the Cardiology Section of the Department of Medicine, East Carolina University School of Medicine, March 1991.

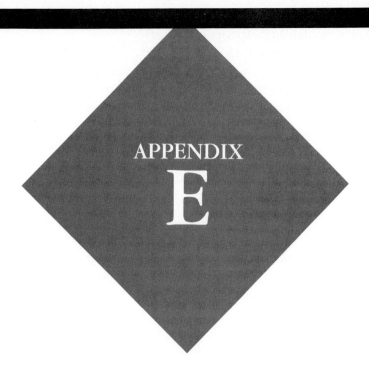

APPENDIX E

Documentation

BARRY BUNN, EMT-P

Objectives

A paramedic should be able to—

1. Define the following terms relevant to documentation:
   a. Anatomic figure, injury identification
   b. Chief complaint (CC)
   c. Demographic information
   d. History of present illness/injury (HPI)
   e. Past medical history (PMH)
   f. Pertinent negatives
   g. Pertinent positives
   h. Physician orders
   i. Response to treatment
   j. Review of systems (ROS)/physical assessment
   k. Treatment

2. Using an acceptable format, demonstrate proper documentation.

Documentation is often considered the evil part of any healthcare professional's job, and emergency medical service (EMS) professionals are no different. Emphasis on documentation has increased dramatically, paralleled by sophistication of patient care and rise in medical litigation. Emphasis on documentation can also be attributed to increased quality assessment/improvement, educational levels, and awareness of EMS professionals.

Documentation should be practiced and tested just like any other technical skill. Refining a few definitions and procedures will help to avoid pitfalls, enhance the delivery of patient care, and reduce the risk of litigation. Documentation procedures—

- Provide a record of scene information that may not be available from any other source.
- Provide continuity of care from one healthcare professional to another.
- Provide medicolegal evidence.
- Reveal any significant changes in the patient's condition.
- Provide an internal tool for statistics, budgeting, and quality assessment/improvement.
- Reveal problems with record-keeping procedures.

Procedure

1. Collect all patient demographic information (e.g., name, age, sex, address).

2. Complete all blanks and check all pertinent boxes on the call report form.

3. Begin the narrative by documenting the patient's level of consciousness (LOC), age, and how he or she appears initially. "20 y.o. male found supine on living room floor, conscious and alert."

4. Document patient's chief complaint. This should be in the patient's own words and included in quotation marks, if possible.

5. Document history of present illness. This should be given in chronologic sequence and should include the time of onset, frequency, lo-

Definitions

Anatomic figure, injury identification is an anterior and posterior figure located on the call report form. It should be used to mark and label the patient's injuries.

Chief complaint (CC) is a brief sentence or statement describing the patient's reason for seeking medical attention. It should be the patient's own words if possible (e.g, "My chest hurts" or "I can't catch my breath").

Demographic data include name, age, date of birth, address, occupation, and nearest relative.

History of present illness/injury (HPI) documents events or complaints associated with the patient's deviation from normal health. This should correlate with the reason the person is seeking medical attention only for his or her current medical problem, not past problems (e.g., "While painting last night around 10:00 PM, I began having this dull pain in my chest" or "I lost control of my motorcycle and slid about 50 feet down the roadway").

Past medical history (PMH) documents any significant past medical or traumatic illnesses that relate to the patient's present illness or injury. These data should include hospitalizations, surgeries, illnesses, or injuries.

Pertinent negative is the absence of a sign or symptom that helps to substantiate or identify a patient's condition. For example, a patient with a suspected dislocated hip usually has decreased range of motion; if the patient has good range of motion, this should be documented.

Pertinent positive is the presence of a sign or symptom that helps to substantiate or identify a patient's condition. For example, if a patient falls and complains of leg pain, an obvious bend of the midshaft lower leg is a positive sign of injury and should be documented.

Physician orders are physician-directed advanced life support (ALS) or basic life support (BLS) treatment orders.

Response to treatment is the patient's response or lack of response to the care that was rendered.

Review of systems (ROS)/physical assessment are two separate categories that should be combined in the EMS field assessment. The review of systems is a head-to-toe review of all complaints system-by-system. The physical assessment is a head-to-toe, hands-on examination. These two should be combined for EMS documentation into the complaints and physical findings.

Treatment is the care rendered to the patient.

cation, quantity, character of the problem, setting, and anything that aggravates or alleviates the problem.

6. Document review systems and physical assessment findings, including any pertinent positives or negatives. This should be a head-to-toe assessment, when indicated.

7. Document any significant past medical history, including surgeries, hospitalizations, illnesses, or injuries.

8. Document allergies and current medications.

9. Document treatment procedures, who performed the procedures, and the patient's response or lack of response to treatment. Include times.

10. Document vital signs and orders, with times.

11. Attach all EKG strips documented with date, time, lead, and patient's name.

12. Complete Glasgow Coma Scale, with times.

13. Complete Trauma Score, if indicated.

14. Complete injury location chart, if indicated.

15. Obtain receiving nurse's and doctor's signature as needed.

16. Leave copy of report with patient's chart.

PEARLS & PITFALLS

Additional Documentation Tips

1. Do not blacken through any documentation; draw one line through it and place your initials beside it.
2. Use correct spelling.
3. If normal protocol or standard of care was not followed, document why.
4. Document any delays or problems responding, gaining access, or transporting the patient. Include an explanation of the problem and the length of the delay.
5. Document any domestic problems that might have arisen.
6. Use a supplement sheet when necessary. The narrative does not have to be squeezed into a small area on the call report form.
7. Use approved medical abbreviations.
8. Write legibly, clearly, and concisely.
9. A patient who presents with trauma and has experienced a significant mechanism of injury should have a documented head-to-toe physical assessment, not just of areas of major complaint.
10. Complete the form as soon as possible; it enhances accuracy.
11. REMEMBER, IF IT WAS NOT DOCUMENTED, IT WAS NOT DONE!

Documentation by Call Type

The following lists are specific pieces of information that may be necessary for complete and accurate documentation. This information is not in prioritized order. These lists indicate suggested items that should be included in your documentation.

Car crash

- Patient location in auto
- Seatbelt or shoulder harness usage
- Loss of consciousness
- Velocity of accident
- Type of accident (head-on, roll-over)
- Type of vehicle damage
- Patient trapped or pinned
- Delay in extrication
- Patient ejected from vehicle
- Patient ambulatory at scene

Chest pain

- Activity at time of pain onset
- Radiation
- Pain on movement
- Onset (gradual or sudden)
- Breath sounds (presence, quality, and quantity)
- Dyspnea
- Nausea and/or vomiting
- Diaphoresis
- Jugular venous distention
- Peripheral edema
- Pain character (sharp, dull)

For any type of pain, the PQRST format can be used: P—Provokes, Q—Quality, R—Radiates, S—Severity, and T—Time

Coma

- Sign or history of trauma
- History of diabetes or seizure
- Drug or alcohol ingestion
- Last seen conscious by whom and when
- Position found
- Scene survey
- Pupils
- Response to painful or verbal stimulus

Diabetes

- Level of consciousness
- Insulin-dependent or oral hypoglycemics
- Last meal
- Amount of exercise
- Last insulin injection and how much
- Any recent illnesses
- Gradual or rapid onset of symptoms
- Kussmaul breathing
- Alcohol or other drug use

Gunshot wound

- Number of wounds
- Location of wounds
- Type of weapon (handgun, rifle, or shotgun)
- Patient's position at time of shooting
- Perpetrator's position at time of shooting
- How many shots heard
- Head-to-toe assessment
- Note caliber of weapon, if it can be confirmed
- Amount of external hemorrhage noted
- Police notification

No transport call

- Clear documentation
- Patient demographic information
- Patient informed of consequences of not being transported
- Methods used to encourage patient to accept treatment/transportation
- Alcohol or other drug usage
- Level of consciousness
- Patient's reason for contacting EMS
- Individual responsible for contacting EMS, if not the patient
- Vital signs
- Physical exam
- Cancellations en route noted (e.g., police, fire, dispatch)
- Patient's cooperation with your attempt to deliver care and transport
- Signature of patient
- Signature of witnesses

Documentation by Call Type—cont'd

Overdose

- Level of consciousness
- Whether overdose was witnessed or not
- Medication or substance ingested
- Amount ingested
- Time of overdose or best approximation
- Any associated alcohol or drug consumption
- Prior overdose or suicide attempts
- Patient admission of intent to harm self
- Police notification

Pediatric

- Level of consciousness (crying, uninterested)
- Parent recognition
- Consolable
- Head bob
- Fontanelles (full, flat, or sunken)
- Child's weight
- Skin condition
- Sucking reflex
- Finger grasp
- Response to pain
- Fever
- Length of illness
- Medications or treatments administered

Pregnancy

- Last menstrual period
- Estimated due date (if known)
- Number of pregnancies (gravida)
- Number of pregnancies carried to term (para)
- Prenatal care history (none, some, continuous)
- Complications with this pregnancy
- Complications with other pregnancies
- Water broke
- Back pain
- Urge to push
- Vaginal discharge
- Multiple births
- Type of pain
- Duration of pain
- Regularity of pain
- Interval between pains
- Progress during transport

Respiratory distress

- Level of consciousness
- Skin color and temperature
- Amount of distress (mild, moderate, or severe)
- Audible respiratory sounds (wheezes, rales, rhonchi)
- Onset of distress (gradual or sudden)
- Activity at time of onset
- Cardiac history
- COPD history
- Breath sounds (present, absent, wheezes, rales)

Seizure

- Level of consciousness
- History of seizures
- History of alcohol or other drug usage
- History of diabetes
- Sign or history of injury
- Number of seizures
- Duration of seizures
- Motor activity observed during seizure (e.g., where began and spread)
- Medication history (i.e., takes seizure or diabetic medications regularly)
- Pupils
- Breath sounds
- Head-to-toe assessment
- Cardiac history

Stab wounds

- Number of wounds
- Location of wounds
- Amount of external hemorrhage noted
- Patient's position at time of stabbing
- Perpetrator's position and knife angle at time of stabbing
- Head-to-toe assessment
- Scene survey
- Police notification

Trauma

- Level of consciousness
- Type of accident
- Ambulatory after accident
- Head-to-toe assessment
- Special circumstances
- Scene survey

Documentation

Procedure	Possible points	Points awarded
Obtain demographic information.	1	
Clearly define chief complaint.	1	
Note initial level of consciousness.	1	
Define location/presentation.	1	
Obtain history of present illness.	1	
Perform complete physical assessment.	1	
Note pertinent positives.	1	
Note pertinent negatives.	1	
Note pertinent past medical history.	1	
Document allergies.	1	
List current medications.	1	
Record treatment.	1	
Record response to treatment.	1	
Place EKG strip.	1	
Document orders.	1	
Document times.	1	
Record vital signs.	1	
Complete Glasgow Coma Scale.	1	
Completed Trauma Score (if indicated).	1	
Obtain appropriate signatures at receiving facility.	1	
TOTAL POINTS	**20**	

COMMENTS _____

_____

_____

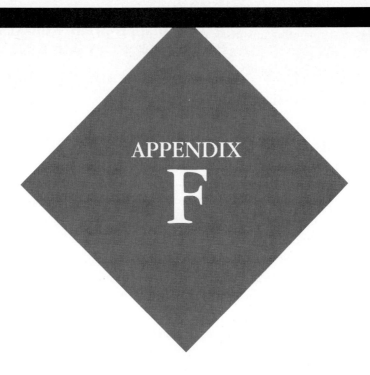

APPENDIX
F

Radio Communications

BARRY BUNN, EMT-P

Objectives

A paramedic should be able to—

1. Demonstrate proper radio presentation of the non-advanced life support (ALS) patient.

2. Demonstrate how to request ALS treatment via the radio.

3. Be able to name factors that affect the approval of ALS orders.

4. Be able to list the components necessary to properly present non-ALS and ALS patients via the radio.

Radio presentation of patient data is not just a technical skill but an art. The development of this skill is often covered briefly in training courses and is rarely tested. Lack of training and testing forces new EMS personnel to learn and develop their radio presentation skills by watching and listening to other EMS personnel. This on-the-job training is an excellent way to learn; however, it may leave many training deficits and bad habits unaddressed.

Numerous EMS personnel find that many of their colleagues have no problem receiving sophisticated ALS treatment orders. Yet, they remain puzzled over the difficulty they have receiving basic ALS treatment orders. This section addresses some of these lingering problems, but the main focus is centered around the assimilation, practice, testing, and transmission of patient data via the radio.

◆ Radio Transmission of the Non-ALS Patient

Non-ALS patients include nonemergent patients whom EMS personnel are transporting to a medical facility. EMS personnel are not requesting orders for the treatment of these patients, but they are transmitting basic patient information to the medical facility. The reason for this transmission is to enable the medical facility to prepare for or triage these patients. This type of transmission should be brief and concise and include basic information.

Procedure

1. Make sure the channel is clear and available for transmission.

2. Depress the push to talk button (PTT) and hold for 1 second.

3. Speak clearly and do not hold the handset too close to your mouth.

4. Call the medical facility and close with your unit number (i.e., "Jones hospital, this is Mercy EMS No. 4").

5. When the hospital responds, give your name, unit, and type of transport traffic (i.e., "Jones, this is Smith on Mercy EMS No. 4, en route, nonemergency traffic").

6. State—
  a. Patient age.
  b. Sex.
  c. Level of consciousness.
  d. Chief complaint.
  e. Brief HPI.
  f. Vital signs (V/S) optional.
  g. Patient assessment.
  h. Treatment.
  i. Estimated time of arrival (ETA).

7. Listen for the hospital's response, which may include room assignment or further disposition.

8. Acknowledge the receipt of that information and clear the channel.

Inappropriate Non-ALS Transmission

EMS: Jones Hospital, this is Mercy EMS No. 4 calling.

Hospital: This is Jones Hospital, Mercy EMS No. 4.

EMS: We are en route nonemergency, with a 20-year-old patient who lost control of his bicycle, landing on the roadway. The patient was found walking around at the scene complaining of pain to the inferior aspect of the right shoulder, and pain to the right lateral malleolus and the palmar aspect of the right hand. The patient has bruising with a large abrasion to the right shoulder, a 1-cm superficial laceration to the lateral malleolus with edema, tenderness, and decreased range of motion. The patient also has abrasions to the right hand. We have placed a dressing and frac-pac splint to the right ankle and an adaptic dressing to the shoulder and right hand. A sling was also placed on the right arm. The patient is immobilized on the scoop stretcher with straps. He moves all extremities and denies loss of consciousness. Pupils are equal and reactive to light. Blood pressure is 120/74, pulse is 92 regular, respiration 24 clear. Our ETA is approximately 10 minutes.

Hospital: Mercy EMS No. 4, take your patient to room No. 12.

EMS: Copy, take patient to room No. 12.

Critique

- The report is too wordy.
- It doesn't flow.
- It is easy to lose sight of the chief complaint.
- The report is too descriptive for this type of transmission. This information can be reported on arrival at the hospital and contained within the written documentation.
- Most of this information is not heard or recorded by emergency department personnel.
- The report takes up too much radio time.
- The report did not report anything wrong, just reported too much.

Appropriate Non-ALS Transmission

EMS: Jones Hospital, this is Mercy EMS No. 4 calling.

Hospital: This is Jones Hospital, go ahead Mercy EMS No. 4.

EMS: This is paramedic Smith, on Mercy EMS No. 4, en route nonemergency traffic with a conscious 20-year-old male who fell from his bicycle while riding on the roadway. He was found ambulatory, complaining of pain to the right shoulder, ankle, and hand. He has multiple abrasions and decreased range of motion to the right ankle. He denies loss of consciousness, moves all extremities. Patient is stabilized on scoop stretcher with splint to the right leg and arm. Vital signs within normal limits. ETA approximately 10 minutes.

Hospital: Mercy EMS No. 4, take your patient to room No. 12.

EMS: Copy, take patient to room No. 12.

Critique

- The report flows well.
- It is easy to follow.
- It gives a clear picture, but is not too descriptive.
- The chief complaint is clearly stated.

◆ Radio Transmission of the ALS Patient

ALS patients include all patients who require direct physician contact to receive ALS treatment orders, which may include IVs, medications, and surgical cricothyrotomy. ALS communication is of the utmost importance to EMS personnel. It is even more important for the patient who needs the advanced level of care that these orders allow. The critical nature of this skill dictates that it not only be emphasized during training, but that it also be tested regularly.

Procedure

1. Request that communications give you a patch if necessary to the facility of choice (i.e., "C-med, Mercy EMS No. 4. Go ahead

Mercy EMS No. 4. Need a patch to Jones Hospital on Med 7").

2. When patch is completed, depress push to talk (PTT) button on handset and hold for one second.

3. Speak clearly and do not hold the handset too close to mouth.

4. Call the medical facility and close with unit number ("Jones Hospital, this is Mercy EMS No. 4").

5. When the hospital responds, ask to speak with a physician reference paramedic orders ("May I speak with a physician reference paramedic orders?")

6. When the physician answers ("This is Dr. Edwards."), respond by repeating the physician's name, followed by your name, title, and unit number and ask the physician if he receives okay. ("Dr. Edwards, this is paramedic Smith on Mercy EMS No. 4, can you hear me okay?")

7. Give your location on scene or en route, followed by your ETA. ("I'm on the scene approximately 20 minutes from your facility.")

8. If you are en route give transport traffic (emergency or nonemergency).

9. Give patient's age, level of consciousness, and initial presentation.

10. Give patient's chief complaint and a brief concise history of present illness.

11. Give brief, concise, and significant physical assessment findings.

12. Give significant past medical history, accompanied by allergies and medications.

13. Describe treatment already performed and patient's response to treatment.

14. Request desired orders.

15. Repeat orders given by physician.

16. Recontact if transport is delayed, if there is a significant change, or if further orders are desired.

Inappropriate ALS Transmission

EMS: C-med, Mercy EMS No. 4.

Communications: Go ahead Mercy EMS No. 4.

EMS: We need a patch to Jones Hospital on Med 7.

Communications: Mercy EMS No. 4, your patch is complete, call direct.

EMS: Jones Hospital, this is Mercy EMS No. 4.

Hospital: Mercy EMS No. 4, this is Jones Hospital, go ahead.

EMS: I need to speak with a physician reference paramedic orders.

Hospital: Stand by for Dr. Edwards. This is Dr. Edwards, go ahead.

EMS: Dr. Edwards, this is Mercy EMS No. 4, can you hear me okay?

Hospital: I hear you fine, go ahead.

EMS: We have a 50-year-old male. He was found seated on the edge of his bed. He looks pale and sweaty. He is nauseated, but has not vomited. He has some moderate difficulty in breathing. He denies cough or fever. He complains of substernal chest pain that feels like someone is squeezing him. The pain stays in the center of his chest. It does not hurt when he moves. His pupils are equal and reactive to light. He has no postural change in his blood pressure. His lungs are clear, and sounds are present throughout. His conjunctiva is pink. He has no jugular vein distention or peripheral edema. His abdomen or chest is without pain on palpation. He denies any past medical history. He takes no medications and has no allergies.

We put him on the monitor, and it is showing a normal sinus rhythm with multifocal PVCs. His vital signs supine are B/P 110/70, P-88 irregular, R-24 and slightly labored. Vital signs seated upright are B/P 110/70, P-88 irregular, R-24 and slightly labored. He is seated upright on stretcher. We have him on oxygen at 6 L/min via nasal cannula and have started an IV of D_5W at KVO rate in the dorsum of right hand with an 18-gauge catheter. He states his pain is unchanged.

I would like to administer one 1/150 SL nitro every 5 minutes up to three, 100 mg lidocaine intravenously, followed by a 4:1 lidocaine drip to run at 2 mg/min.

Hospital: Go ahead with your nitro and lidocaine, recontact if any change.

EMS: 10-4, Mercy EMS No. 4, clear.

Hospital: Jones Hospital, clear.

Critique

- Paramedic did not report ETA.
- Report does not flow and is too wordy.
- The wordiness clouds the chief complaint.
- Unnecessary information is reported (e.g., type of IV and site)
- The report takes up too much radio time.
- The paramedic did not repeat orders so physician could validate.
- The paramedic did not give his or her name or title at the beginning of the transmission.

Appropriate ALS Transmission

EMS: C-med, Mercy EMS No. 4.

Communications: Go ahead, Mercy EMS No. 4.

EMS: We need a patch to Jones Hospital on Med 7.

Communications: Mercy EMS No. 4, your patch is complete, call direct.

EMS: Jones Hospital, this is Mercy EMS No. 4.

Hospital: Mercy EMS No. 4, this is Jones Hospital, go ahead.

EMS: I need to speak with a physician reference paramedic orders.

Hospital: Stand by for Dr. Edwards. This is Dr. Edwards, go ahead.

EMS: Dr. Edwards, this is paramedic Smith on Mercy EMS No. 4, can you hear me okay?

Hospital: I hear you fine, go ahead.

EMS: We are at the scene approximately 20 minutes from your facility with a 50-year-old male who is conscious, alert, pale, and sweaty. Patient stated he awoke from his sleep approximately 20 minutes ago with severe, squeezing, nonradiating chest pain. His pain is accompanied by moderate dyspnea, diaphoresis, nausea, but no vomiting. The pain is constant and unchanged by movement or palpation. Physical exam reveals lungs clear throughout, no jugular venous distention, and no peripheral edema. He denies any significant past medical history, takes no medications, and has no allergies. The monitor is showing normal sinus rhythm with approximately 12 multifocal PVCs per minute. B/P 110/70, P-88, irregular R-24.

We are administering oxygen at 6 L/min via nasal cannula, and we have initiated an IV D_5W KVO.

I would like to administer nitroglycerin one 1/150 SL q 5 minutes up to three, lidocaine 100 mg IV, followed by a 4:1 lidocaine drip at 2 mg/min.

Hospital: Go ahead with your nitroglycerin and lidocaine, recontact with any change.

EMS: Confirming nitroglycerin one 1/150 SL q 5 minutes up to three, lidocaine 100 mg IV, followed by a 4:1 lidocaine drip at 2 mg/min.

Hospital: 0-4. Jones Hospital clear.

EMS: Mercy EMS No. 4 clear.

Critique
- Transmission is orderly.
- It is clear and easy to follow.
- The parmedic gives only pertinent data and excludes extraneous information.
- The transmission does not take too much radio time.
- The paramedic repeats orders for physician to validate.
- The paramedic reports ETA.

◆ Factors that Affect the Approval of ALS Orders
- Physician preference
- Hospital variances
- EMS personnel's reputation and credibility
- Deficit of assessment skills
- Lack of confidence
- Knowledge deficit, related to treatment regimens
- Transmission too wordy
- Omission of critical information
- Poor radio quality during transmission
- Vocabulary of ALS personnel
- Verbal communication skills deficit
- Short transport time

ALS Radio Transmission

Procedure	Possible points	Points awarded
Depress microphone key.	1	
Request communications patch to medical facility.	1	
Request to speak with physician for paramedic orders.	1	
Begin transmission by repeating physician's name.	1	
Give technician's name, title, and unit.	1	
Give patient's age and sex.	2	
Give level of consciousness.	1	
Give chief complaint.	1	
Give initial presentation.	1	
Give brief appropriate history of present illness (HPI).	1	
Describe brief, concise, and significant physical assessment findings.	1	
Give significant past medical history.	1	
Give allergies and current medications.	2	
Describe treatment given.	1	
Describe response to treatment.	1	
Request appropriate orders.	1	
Listen and repeat physician's order.	1	
Give estimated time of arrival.	1	
TOTAL POINTS	**20**	

COMMENTS _____

_____

_____

Non-ALS Radio Transmission

Procedure	Possible points	Points awarded
Depress microphone key.	1	
Speak clearly.	1	
Give medical facility name, followed by unit name and number.	1	
Give name, unit, and transport traffic.	1	
Give patient age and sex.	1	
Give level of consciousness.	1	
Give chief complaint.	1	
Give brief appropriate history of present illness (HPI) and vital signs.	2	
Describe physical assessment findings	1	
Describe treatment given.	1	
Describe response to treatment.	1	
Request appropriate orders.	1	
Listen and repeat physician's order.	1	
Give estimated time of arrival.	1	
TOTAL POINTS	**15**	

COMMENTS _____

_____

_____

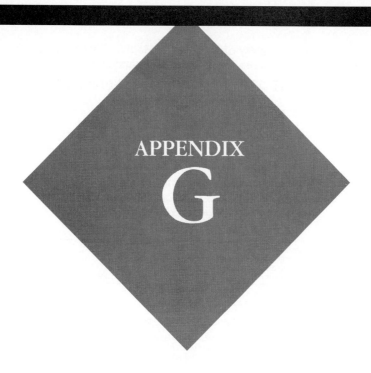

APPENDIX
G

National Registry of
EMT-Paramedic Examination
Skill Sheets

(Courtesy The National Registry of Emergency Medical Technicians, Columbus, Ohio; 1992)

National Registry of Emergency Medical Technicians
Advanced Level Practical Examination
PATIENT ASSESSMENT/MANAGEMENT

Candidate:_____   Examiner:_____

Date._____   Signature:_____

Scenario #_____   Time Start:_____Time End:_____

PRIMARY SURVEY/RESUSCITATION

		Possible Points	Points Awarded
Takes or verbalizes infection control precautions		1	
Airway with C-Spine Control	Takes or directs manual in-line immobilization of head (1 point) Opens and assesses airway (1 point) Inserts adjunct (1 point)	3	
Breathing	Assesses breathing (1 point) Initiates appropriate oxygen therapy (1 point) Assures adequate ventilation of patient (1 point) Manages any injury which may compromise breathing/ventilation (1 point)	4	
Circulation	Checks pulse (1 point) Assesses peripheral perfusion (1 point) [checks either skin color, temperature, or capillary refill] Assesses for and controls major bleeding if present (1 point) Takes vital signs (1 point) Verbalizes application of or consideration for PASG (1 point) [candidate must assess body parts to be enclosed prior to application]	5	
	Volume replacement [usually deferred until patient loaded] - Initiates first IV line (1 point) - Initiates second IV line (1 point) - Selects appropriate catheters (1 point) - Selects appropriate IV solutions and administration sets (1 point) - Infuses at appropriate rate (1 point)	5	
Disability	Performs mini-neuro assessment: AVPU (1 point) Applies cervical collar (1 point)	2	
Expose	Removes clothing	1	
Status	Calls for immediate transport of the patient when indicated	1	

PRIMARY SURVEY/RESUSCITATION SUB-TOTAL   22

SECONDARY SURVEY

NOTE: Areas denoted by **** may be integrated within sequence of Primary Survey

		Possible Points	Points Awarded
Head	Inspects mouth**, nose**, and assesses facial area (1 point) Inspects and palpates scalp and ears (1 point) Checks eyes: PEARRL** (1 point)	3	
Neck**	Checks position of trachea (1 point) Checks jugular veins (1 point) Palpates cervical spine (1 point)	3	
Chest**	Inspects chest (1 point) Palpates chest (1 point) Auscultates chest (1 point)	3	
Abdomen/Pelvis**	Inspects and palpates abdomen (1 point) Assesses pelvis (1 point)	2	
Lower Extremities**	Inspects and palpates left leg (1 point) Inspects and palpates right leg (1 point) Checks motor, sensory, and distal circulation (1 point/leg)	4	
Upper Extremities	Inspects and palpates left arm (1 point) Inspects and palpates right arm (1 point) Checks motor, sensory, and distal circulation (1 point/arm)	4	
Posterior Thorax/Lumbar** and Buttocks	Inspects and palpates posterior thorax (1 point) Inspects and palpates lumbar and buttocks area (1 point)	2	
Identifies and treats minor wounds/fractures appropriately (1 point each)		2	

SECONDARY SURVEY SUB-TOTAL   23

CRITICAL CRITERIA
____ Failure to initiate or call for transport of the patient within 10 minute time limit
____ Failure to take or verbalize infection control precautions
____ Failure to immediately establish and maintain spinal protection
____ Failure to provide high concentration of oxygen
____ Failure to evaluate and find all presented conditions of airway, breathing, and circulation (shock)
____ Failure to appropriately manage/provide airway, breathing, hemorrhage control or treatment for shock
____ Failure to differentiate patient's needing transportation versus continued on-scene survey
____ Does other detailed physical examination before assessing & treating threats to airway, breathing & circulation

You must factually document your rationale for checking any of the above critical items on the reverse side of this form.

National Registry of Emergency Medical Technicians
Paramedic Practical Examination
VENTILATORY MANAGEMENT (ET)

Candidate:_____   Examiner:_____

Date:_____   Signature:_____

NOTE: If canditate elects to initially ventilate with BVM attached to reservoir and oxygen, full credit must
be awarded for steps denoted by "***" so long as first ventilation is delivered within initial 30 seconds.

	Possible Points	Points Awarded
Takes or verbalizes infection control precautions	1	
Opens the airway manually	1	
Elevates tongue, inserts simple adjunct [either oropharyngeal or nasopharyngeal airway]	1	
NOTE: Examiner now informs candidate no gag reflex is present and patient accepts adjunct		
**Ventilates patient immediately with bag-valve-mask device unattached to oxygen	1	
**Hyperventilates patient with room air	1	
NOTE: Examiner now informs candidate that ventilation is being performed without difficulty		
Attaches oxygen reservoir to bag-valve-mask device and connects to high flow oxygen regulator [12-15 liters/min.]	1	
Ventilates patient at a rate of 12-20/min. and volumes of at least 800ml	1	
NOTE: After 30 seconds, examiner auscultates and reports breath sounds are present and equal bilaterally and medical control has ordered intubation. The examiner must now take over ventilation.		
Directs assistant to hyperventilate patient	1	
Identifies/selects proper equipment for intubation	1	
Checks equipment for: - Cuff leaks (1 point) - Laryngoscope operational and bulb tight (1 point)	2	
NOTE: Examiner to remove OPA and move out of way when candidate is prepared to intubate		
Positions head properly	1	
Inserts blade while displacing tongue	1	
Elevates mandible with laryngoscope	1	
Introduces ET tube and advances to proper depth	1	
Inflates cuff to proper pressure and disconnects syringe	1	
Directs ventilation of patient	1	
Confirms proper placement by auscultation bilaterally and over epigastrium	1	
NOTE: Examiner to ask "If you had proper placement, what would you expect to hear?"		
Secures ET tube [may be verbalized]	1	

CRITICAL CRITERIA   **TOTAL** 19 [   ]

____ Failure to initiate ventilations within 30 seconds after applying gloves or interrupts ventilations
       for greater than 30 seconds at any time

____ Failure to take or verbalize infection control precautions

____ Failure to voice and ultimately provide high oxygen concentrations [at least 85%]

____ Failure to ventilate patient at rate of at least 12/minute

____ Failure to provide adequate volumes per breath [maximum 2 errors/minute permissable]

____ Failure to hyperventilate patient prior to intubation

____ Failure to successfully intubate within 3 attempts

____ Using teeth as a fulcrum

____ Failure to assure proper tube placement by auscultation bilaterally **and** over the epigastrium

____ If used, stylette extends beyond end of ET tube

____ Inserts any adjunct in a manner dangerous to patient

You must factually document your rationale for checking any of the above critical items on the reverse side of this form.

National Registry of Emergency Medical Technicians
Intermediate Practical Examination
VENTILATORY MANAGEMENT (EOA)

Candidate:_____ Examiner:_____

Date:_____ Signature:_____

NOTE: If canditate elects to initially ventilate with BVM attached to reservoir and oxygen, full credit must be awarded for steps denoted by "**" so long as first ventilation is delivered within initial 30 seconds.

	Possible Points	Points Awarded
Takes or verbalizes infection control precautions	1	
Opens the airway manually	1	
Elevates tongue, inserts simple adjunct [either oropharyngeal or nasopharyngeal airway]	1	
NOTE: Examiner now informs candidate no gag reflex is present and patient accepts adjunct		
**Ventilates patient immediately with bag-valve-mask device unattached to oxygen	1	
**Hyperventilates patient with room air	1	
NOTE: Examiner now informs candidate that ventilation is being performed without difficulty		
Attaches oxygen reservoir to bag-valve-mask device and connects to high flow oxygen regulator [12-15 liters/min.]	1	
Ventilates patient at a rate of 12-20/min. and volumes of at least 800ml	1	
NOTE: After 30 seconds, examiner auscultates and reports breath sounds are present and equal bilaterally and medical control has ordered placement of an EOA. The examiner must now take over ventilation.		
Directs assistant to hyperventilate patient	1	
Identifies/selects proper equipment	1	
Assembles airway	1	
Tests cuff	1	
Inflates mask	1	
Lubricates tube [may be verbalized]	1	
NOTE: Examiner to remove OPA and move out of way when candidate is prepared to insert EOA		
Positions head properly with neck in neutral or slightly flexed position	1	
Grasps tongue and mandible and elevates	1	
Inserts tube in same direction as curvature of pharynx	1	
Advances tube until mask sealed against face	1	
Ventilates patient while maintaining tight mask seal	1	
Directs confirmation of proper placement by auscultation bilaterally and over epigastrium	1	
Inflates cuff to proper pressure and disconnects syringe	1	
Continues ventilation of patient	1	
NOTE: Examiner to ask "If you had proper placement, what would you expect to hear?"		

TOTAL 21 [ ]

CRITICAL CRITERIA

___ Failure to initiate ventilations within 30 seconds after applying gloves or interrupts ventilations for greater than 30 seconds at any time

___ Failure to take or verbalize infection control precautions

___ Failure to voice and ultimately provide high oxygen concentrations [at least 85%]

___ Failure to ventilate patient at rate of at least 12/minute

___ Failure to provide adequate volumes per breath [maximum 2 errors/minute permissable]

___ Failure to hyperventilate patient prior to placement of the EOA

___ Failure to successfully place the EOA within 3 attempts

___ Failure to assure proper tube placement by auscultation bilaterally **and** over the epigastrium

___ Inserts any adjunct in a manner dangerous to patient

You must factually document your rationale for checking any of the above critical items on the reverse side of this form.

National Registry of Emergency Medical Technicians
Paramedic Practical Examination
CARDIAC ARREST SKILLS STATION
DYNAMIC CARDIOLOGY

Candidate:_____   Examiner:_____

Date:_____   Signature:_____

Set #_____   Time Start:_____Time End:_____

	Possible Points	Points Awarded
Takes or verbalizes infection control precautions	1	
Checks level of responsiveness	1	
Checks ABC's	1	
Initiates CPR if appropriate [verbally]	1	
Performs "Quick Look" with paddles	1	
Correctly interprets initial rhythm	1	
Appropriately manages initial rhythm	2	
Notes change in rhythm	1	
Checks patient condition to include pulse and, if appropriate, BP	1	
Correctly interprets second rhythm	1	
Appropriately manages second rhythm	2	
Notes change in rhythm	1	
Checks patient condition to include pulse and, if appropriate, BP	1	
Correctly interprets third rhythm	1	
Appropriately manages third rhythm	2	
Notes change in rhythm	1	
Checks patient condition to include pulse and, if appropriate, BP	1	
Correctly interprets fourth rhythm	1	
Appropriately manages fourth rhythm	2	
Orders high percentages of supplemental oxygen at proper times	1	

CRITICAL CRITERIA   **TOTAL** 24 [ ]

____ Failure to deliver first shock in a timely manner due to operator delay in machine use or providing treatments
　　　 other than CPR with simple adjuncts
____ Failure to deliver second or third shocks without delay other than the time required to reassess and recharge paddles
____ Failure to order or perform pulse checks before and after shocks
____ Failure to ensure the safety of self and others [verbalizes"All clear" and observes]
____ Inability to deliver DC shock [does not use machine properly]
____ Failure to demonstrate acceptable shock sequence
____ Failure to order initiation or resumption of CPR when appropriate
____ Failure to order correct management of airway [ET when appropriate]
____ Failure to order administration of appropriate oxygen at proper time
____ Failure to diagnose or treat 2 or more rhythms correctly
____ Orders administration of an inappropriate drug or lethal dosage
____ Failure to correctly diagnose or adequately treat v-fib, v-tach, or asystole

You must factually document your rationale for checking any of the above critical items on the reverse side of this form.

National Registry of Emergency Medical Technicians
Paramedic Practical Examination
CARDIAC ARREST SKILLS STATION
STATIC CARDIOLOGY

Candidate:_____   Examiner:_____

Date:_____ _____   Signature:_____

Set #_____

NOTE: No points for treatment may be awarded if the diagnosis is incorrect.
       Only document incorrect responses in spaces provided.

	Points Awarded	Possible Points
STRIP #1		
Diagnosis:	1	
Treatment:	2	
STRIP #2		
Diagnosis:	1	
Treatment:	2	
STRIP #3		
Diagnosis:	1	
Treatment:	2	
STRIP #4		
Diagnosis:	1	
Treatment:	2	
TOTAL	12	

National Registry of Emergency Medical Technicians
Advanced Level Practical Examination
INTRAVENOUS THERAPY

Candidate:_____   Examiner:_____

Date:_____   Signature:_____

Time Start:_____Time End:_____

	Possible Points	Points Awarded

Checks selected IV fluid for:
    - Proper fluid (1 point)
    - Clarity (1 point)
	2	

Selects appropriate catheter	1	
Selects proper administration set	1	
Connects IV tubing to the IV bag	1	
Prepares administration set [fills drip chamber and flushes tubing]	1	
Cuts or tears tape [at any time before venipuncture]	1	
Takes/verbalizes infection control precautions [prior to venipuncture]	1	
Applies tourniquet	1	
Palpates suitable vein	1	
Cleanses site appropriately	1	

Performs venipuncture
 	
    - Inserts stylette (1 point)
    - Notes or verbalizes flashback (1 point)
    - Occludes vein proximal to catheter (1 point)
    - Removes stylette (1 point)
    - Connects IV tubing to catheter (1 point)
	5	

Releases tourniquet	1	
Runs IV for a brief period to assure patent line	1	
Secures catheter [tapes securely or verbalizes]	1	
Adjusts flow rate as appropriate	1	
Disposes/verbalizes disposal of needle in proper container	1	

TOTAL 21 [ ]

CRITICAL CRITERIA

___ Exceeded the 6 minute time limit in establishing a patent and properly adjusted IV

___ Failure to take or verbalize infection control precautions prior to performing venipuncture

___ Contaminates equipment or site without appropriately correcting situation

___ Any improper technique resulting in the potential for catheter shear or air embolism

___ Failure to successfully establish IV within 3 attempts during 6 minute time limit

___ Failure to dispose/verbalize disposal of needle in proper container

You must factually document your rationale for checking any of the above critical items on the reverse side of this form.

National Registry of Emergency Medical Technicians
Paramedic Practical Examination
INTRAVENOUS BOLUS MEDICATIONS

Candi-
date:_____   Examiner:_____

Date:_____   Signature:_____

Time Start:_____Time End:_____

NOTE: Check here (_____) if candidate did not establish
a patent IV and do not evaluate these skills.

	Possible Points	Points Awarded
Asks patient for known allergies	1	
Selects correct medication	1	
Assures correct concentration of drug	1	
Assembles prefilled syringe correctly and dispels air	1	
Continues infection control precautions	1	
Cleanses injection site (Y-port or hub)	1	
Reaffirms medication	1	
Stops IV flow (pinches tubing)	1	
Administers correct dose at proper push rate	1	
Flushes tubing (runs wide open for a brief period)	1	
Adjusts drip rate to TKO (KVO)	1	
Voices proper disposal of syringe and needle	1	
Verbalizes need to observe patient for desired effect/adverse side effects	1	

CRITICAL CRITERIA   IV BOLUS SUB-TOTAL   13   [   ]

___Failure to begin administration of medication within 3 minute time limit

___Contaminates equipment or site without appropriately correcting situation

___Failure to adequately dispel air resulting in potential for air embolism

___Injects improper drug or dosage (wrong drug, incorrect amount, or pushes at inappropriate rate)

___Failure to flush IV tubing after injecting medication

___Recaps needle or failure to dispose/verbalize disposal of syringe and needle in proper container

INTRAVENOUS PIGGYBACK MEDICATIONS

	Possible Points	Points Awarded
Has confirmed allergies by now (award point if previously confirmed)		
Checks selected IV fluid for: - Proper fluid (1 point) - Clarity (1 point)	1 2	
Checks selected medication for: - Clarity (1 point) - Concentration of medication (1 point)	2	
Injects correct amount of medication into IV solution given scenario	1	
Connects appropriate administration set to medication solution	1	
Prepares administration set (fills drip chamber and flushes tubing)	1	
Attaches appropriate needle to administration set	1	
Continues infection control precautions	1	
Cleanses port of primary line	1	
Inserts needle into port without contamination	1	
Adjusts flow rate of secondary line as required	1	
Stops flow of primary line	1	
Securely tapes needle	1	
Verbalizes need to observe patient for desired effect/adverse side effects	1	
Labels medication/fluid bag	1	

CRITICAL CRITERIA   IV PIGGYBACK SUB-TOTAL   17   [   ]

___ Failure to begin administration of medication within 5 minute time limit

___ Contaminates equipment or site without appropriately correcting situation

___ Administers improper drug or dosage (wrong drug, incorrect amount, or infuses at inappropriate rate)

___ Failure to flush IV tubing of secondary line resulting in potential for air embolism

___ Failure to shut-off flow of primary line

You must factually document your rationale for checking any of the above critical items on the reverse side of this form.

National Registry of Emergency Medical Technicians
Advanced Level Practical Examination
SPINAL IMMOBILIZATION
(SEATED PATIENT)

Candidate:_____   Examiner:_____

Date:_____   Signature:_____

Time Start:_____Time End:_____

	Possible Points	Points Awarded
Takes or verbalizes infection control precautions	1	
Directs assistant to place/maintain head in neutral, in-line position	1	
Directs assistant to maintain manual immobilization of head	1	
Assesses motor, sensory, and distal circulation in extremities	1	
Applies appropriately sized extrication collar	1	
Positions the immobilization device behind the patient	1	
Secures device to the patient's torso	1	
Evaluates torso fixation and adjusts as necessary	1	
Evaluates and pads behind the patient's head as necessary	1	
Secures patient's head to the device	1	
Reassesses motor, sensory, and distal circulation in extremities	1	
Verbalizes moving the patient to a long board properly	1	

TOTAL 12 [ ]

CRITICAL CRITERIA

___ Did not immediately direct or take manual immobilization of head

___ Releases or orders release of manual immobilization before it was maintained mechanically

___ Patient manipulated or moved excessively causing potential spinal compromise

___ Did not complete immobilization of the torso prior to immobilizing the head

___ Device moves excessively up, down, left, or right on patient's torso

___ Torso fixation inhibits chest rise resulting in respiratory compromise

___ Head immobilization allows for excessive movement

___ Upon completion of immobilization, head is not in neutral, in-line position

You must factually document your rationale for checking any of the above critical items on the reverse side of this form.

National Registry of Emergency Medical Technicians
Advanced Level Practical Examination
RANDOM BASIC SKILLS
BLEEDING - WOUNDS - SHOCK

Candidate:_____   Examiner:_____

Date:_____   Signature:_____

Time Start:_____Time End:_____

	Possible Points	Points Awarded
Takes or verbalizes infection control precautions	1	
Applies direct pressure to the wound	1	
Elevates the extremity	1	
Applies pressure dressing to the wound	1	
Bandages wound	1	
NOTE: The examiner must now inform the candidate that the wound is still continuing to bleed. The second dressing does not control the bleeding.		
Locates and applies pressure to appropriate arterial pressure point	1	
NOTE: The examiner must indicate that the victim is in compensatory shock.		
Applies high concentration oxygen	1	
Properly positions patient (supine with legs elevated)	1	
Prevents heat loss (covers patient as appropriate)	1	
NOTE: The examiner must indicate that the victim is in profound shock. Medical control has ordered application and inflation of the Pneumatic Anti-shock Garment.		
Removes clothing or checks for sharp objects	1	
Quickly assesses areas that will be under the PASG	1	
Positions PASG with top of abdominal section at or below last set of ribs	1	
Secures PASG around patient	1	
Attaches hoses	1	
Begins inflation sequence (examiner to stop inflation at 15mm Hg)	1	
Checks blood pressure	1	
Verbalizes when to stop inflation sequence	1	
Operates PASG to maintain air pressure in device	1	
Reassesses vital signs	1	

TOTAL 19 [____]

CRITICAL CRITERIA

____ Failure to take or verbalize infection control precautions

____ Did not apply high concentration of oxygen

____ Applies tourniquet before attempting other methods of hemorrhage control

____ Did not control hemorrhage or attempt to control hemorrhage in a timely manner

____ Inflates abdominal section of PASG before the legs

____ Did not reassess patient's vital signs after PASG inflation

____ Places PASG on inside-out

____ Allows deflation of PASG after inflation

____ Positions PASG above level of lowest rib

You must factually document your rationale for checking any of the above critical items on the reverse side of this form.

**National Registry of Emergency Medical Technicians
Advanced Level Practical Examination
RANDOM BASIC SKILLS
LONG BONE IMMOBILIZATION**

Candidate:_____   Examiner:_____

Date:_____   Signature:_____

                                                        Time Start:_____Time End:_____

	Possible Points	Points Awarded
Takes or verbalizes infection control precautions	1	
Directs application of manual stabilization	1	
Assesses motor, sensory, and distal circulation	1	
NOTE: Examiner acknowledges present and normal		
Measures splint	1	
Applies splint	1	
Immobilizes joint above fracture	1	
Immobilizes joint below fracture	1	
Secures entire injured extremity	1	
Immobilizes hand/foot in position of function	1	
Reassesses motor, sensory, and distal circulation	1	
NOTE: Examiner acknowledges present and normal		

TOTAL 10 ☐

CRITICAL CRITERIA

___ Grossly moves injured extremity

___ Did not immobilize adjacent joints, injury, or limb

___ Did not reassess motor, sensory, and distal circulation **after** splinting

You must factually document your rationale for checking any of the above critical items on the reverse side of this form.

National Registry of Emergency Medical Technicians
Advanced Level Practical Examination
RANDOM BASIC SKILLS
TRACTION SPLINTING

Candidate:_____   Examiner:_____

Date:_____   Signature:_____

Time Start:_____Time End:_____

	Possible Points	Points Awarded
Takes or verbalizes infection control precautions	1	
Directs manual stabilization of injured leg	1	
Directs application of manual traction	1	
Assesses motor, sensory, and distal circulation	1	
NOTE: Examiner acknowledges present and normal		
Prepares/adjusts splint to proper length	1	
Positions splint at injured leg	1	
Applies proximal securing device (e.g. ischial strap)	1	
Applies distal securing device (e.g. ankle hitch)	1	
Applies mechanical traction	1	
Positions/secures support straps	1	
Re-evaluates proximal/distal securing devices	1	
Reassesses motor, sensory, and distal circulation	1	
NOTE: Examiner acknowledges present and normal		
NOTE: Examiner must ask candidate how he/she would prepare for transport		
Verbalizes securing torso to long board to immobilize hip	1	
Verbalizes securing splint to long board to prevent movement of splint	1	

TOTAL   14   [ ]

CRITICAL CRITERIA

____ Loss of traction at any point after it is assumed

____ Did not reassess motor, sensory, and distal circulation **after** splinting

____ The foot is excessively rotated or extended after splinting

____ Did not secure ischial strap **before** taking traction

____ Final immobilization failed to support femur or prevent rotation of injured leg

NOTE: If Sagar is used without elevating the leg, application of manual traction is not necessary.
Candidate will be awarded 1 point as if manual traction were applied.

NOTE: If the leg is elevated at all, manual traction must be applied before elevating the leg.
The ankle hitch may be applied before elevating the leg and used to pull manual traction.

You must factually document your rationale for checking any of the above critical items on the reverse side of this form.

National Registry of Emergency Medical Technicians
Advanced Level Practical Examination
RANDOM BASIC SKILLS
SPINAL IMMOBILIZATION
(LYING PATIENT)

Candidate_____   Examiner:_____

Date_____   Signature:_____

Time Start:_____Time End:_____

	Possible Points	Points Awarded
Takes or verbalizes infection control procedures	1	
Directs assistant to move patient's head to the neutral in-line position	1	
Directs assistant to maintain manual immobilization of head	1	
Evaluates motor, sensory, and distal circulation in extremities	1	
Applies cervical collar	1	
Positions immobilization device appropriately	1	
Moves victim onto device without compromising the integrity of the spine	1	
Applies padding to voids between the torso and the board as necessary	1	
Immobilizes torso to the device	1	
Evaluates and pads under the patient's head as necessary	1	
Immobilizes the patient's head to the device	1	
Secures legs to the evice	1	
Secures victims arms to the board	1	
Reassesses motor, sensory, and distal circulation	1	

TOTAL 14 [ ]

CRITICAL CRITERIA

___Did not immediately direct manual immobilization of head

___Orders release of manual immobilization before it was maintained mechanically

___ Did not complete immobilization of the torso prior to immobilizing the head

___ Device excessively moves up, down, left or right on patient's torso

___ Head immobilization allows for excessive movement

___ Head is not immobilized in the neutral in-line position

___ Patient was moved excessively causing potential spinal compromise

___ Did not reassess motor, sensory, and distal circulation after immobilization

You must factually document your rationale for checking any of the above critical items on the reverse side of this form.

EMT-INTERMEDIATE APPLICATION

I am submitting this application to test at

_____ In _____ , ____

(Name of Facility)   City   State

on ____/____/____

Date

No.

DATE RECEIVED

The National Registry of Emergency Medical Technicians®

ALL NON-SHADED AREAS MUST BE COMPLETED IN THEIR ENTIRETY.

WR	DATE	P	F		PRACTICAL	DATE	P	F	R	R1 DATE	P	F	R	R2 DATE	P	F
					Take #1											
					Take #2											
					Take #3											

DATE OF APPLICATION	___ -		HAVE YOU EVER APPLIED FOR EMT-I REGISTRATION BEFORE?	☐ YES ☐ NO	IF YES GIVE DATE	

SOCIAL SECURITY NO. ___ - ___ - ___

NATIONAL REGISTRY EMT-A

EMT NO.

(Include copy of card or certificate)

NAME   LAST   FIRST   INITIAL

HOME ADDRESS   **CITY**

STATE   **COUNTY**   **ZIP CODE**   **SITE**   **BIRTHDATE**

PRIMARY OCCUPATION   EMPLOYED BY   ☐ MALE   ☐ FEMALE

EDUCATION   *(circle highest grade completed)*   H.S.   12   COLLEGE   1   2   3   4   5   6   7   8

► **HAVE YOU EVER BEEN CONVICTED OF A FELONY?**   YES ☐   NO ☐   **IF YES: Please submit with this application** ◄ documentation that describes fully the offense, date of offense, copies of relevant court documents, disposition and current status.

TYPE OF EMT-INTERMEDIATE SERVICE - Please check the following type(s) of service(s) in which you are or will be affiliated with as an EMT-Intermediate:

Fire Dept.	Private	Hospital-Based	3rd Service	Volunteer	U.S. Government
Army	Navy	Air Force	Coast Guard	Other _____ (Please List)	

Will you be paid for your services as an EMT-Intermediate?   Yes ☐   No ☐

APPROVED EMT-I COURSE - Applicant must have completed an approved EMT-I Training Program that equals or exceeds the objectives of the National Standard EMT-I Curriculum. Attach a copy of your course completion certificate or a copy of your current EMT-I card. If your primary EMT-I training program is more than two years old and you hold current state certification as an EMT-I you must document completion of an approved EMT-Basic refresher and 12 hours of Intermediate refresher training within the past two years and attach official documentation to this application.

NAME OF INITIAL TRAINING INSTITUTION OR AGENCY	STREET ADDRESS	STATE	DATE COMPLETED

LENGTH IN HOURS	CLASS—ROOM	CLINICAL	FIELD INTERNSHIP	PHYSICIAN DIRECTOR	INSTRUCTOR/COURSE COORDINATOR

CANDIDATES STATEMENT AND SIGNATURE

I hereby affirm and declare that the above information is true and correct and that any fraudulent entry may be considered a sufficient cause for rejection or subsequent revocation. I further agree to abide by all the rules and regulations of the National Registry of EMT's as promulgated by the Board of Directors, and I hereby authorize the National Registry of EMT's to release my examination scores to the teaching institution/agency and the state office of Emergency Medical Services.

Registration Fee (money order only)	$35.00 first time applicants $35.00 for retakes of written	APPLICANT SIGNATURE

PHYSICIANS STATEMENT AND SIGNATURE

As the Medical Director of EMT-Intermediate training/or EMT-Intermediate operations,

I hereby affirm and declare that the above statements are true and that _____

_____

is of sound character and judgement, and that he/she has completed an approved

EMT-Intermediate training program that equals or exceeds the behavioral objectives of the

National Standard Training Curriculum for EMT-Intermediate.

PHYSICIAN'S NAME (PRINT OR TYPE)

PHYSICIAN'S SIGNATURE

LICENSED TO PRACTICE MEDICINE IN THE STATE OF

LICENSE NO

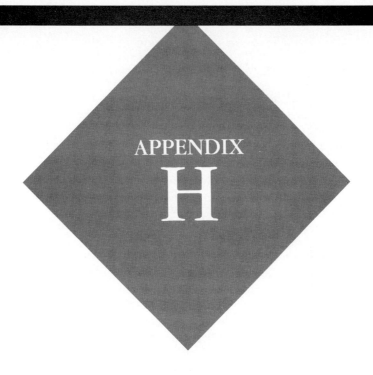

APPENDIX H

American Heart Association Advanced Life Support Algorithms

From American Medical Association: *JAMA* 268:2199-2275, 1992. Copyright 1992, American Medical Association.

Table H-1   The Algorithm Approach to Emergency Cardiac Care

These guidelines use algorithms as an educational tool. They are an illustrative method to summarize information. Providers of emergency care should view algorithms as a summary and a memory aid. They provide a way to treat a broad range of patients. Algorithms, by nature, oversimplify. The effective teacher and care provider will use them wisely, not blindly. Some patients may require care not specified in the algorithms. When clinically appropriate, flexibility is accepted and encouraged. Many interventions and actions are listed as "considerations" to help providers think. These lists should not be considered endorsements or requirements or "standard of care" in a legal sense. Algorithms do not replace clinical understanding. Although the algorithms provide a good "cookbook," the patient always requires a "thinking cook."

The following clinical recommendations apply to all treatment algorithms:

- First, treat the patient, not the monitor.
- Algorithms for cardiac arrest presume that the condition under discussion continually persists, that the patient remains in cardiac arrest, and that CPR is always performed.
- Apply different interventions whenever appropriate indications exist.
- The flow diagrams present mostly Class I (acceptable, definitely effective) recommendations. The footnotes present Class IIa (acceptable, probably effective), Class IIb (acceptable, possibly effective), and Class III (not indicated, may be harmful) recommendations.
- Adequate airway, ventilation, oxygenation, chest compressions, and defibrillation are more important than administration of medications and take precedence over initiating an intravenous line or injecting pharmacologic agents.
- Several medications (epinephrine, lidocaine, and atropine) can be administered via the endotracheal tube, but clinicians must use an endotracheal dose 2 to 2.5 times the intravenous dose.
- With a few exceptions, intravenous medications should always be administered rapidly, in bolus method.
- After each intravenous medication, give a 20- to 30-ml bolus of intravenous fluid and immediately elevate the extremity. This will enhance delivery of drugs to the central circulation, which may take to 1 to 2 minutes.
- Last, treat the patient, not the monitor.

Table H-2   Drugs Used in Pediatric Advanced Life Support*

Drug	Dose	Remarks
Adenosine	0.1 to 0.2 mg/kg Maximum single dose: 12 mg	Rapid IV bolus
Atropine sulfate	0.02 mg/kg per dose	Minimum dose: 0.1 mg Maximum single dose: 0.5 mg in child, 1.0 mg in adolescent
Bretylium	5 mg/kg; may be increased to 10 mg/kg	Rapid IV
Calcium chloride 10%	20 mg/kg per dose	Give slowly
Dopamine hydrochloride	2-20 µg/kg per minute	α-Adrenergic action dominates at ≥ 15-20 µg/kg per minute
Dobutamine hydrochloride	2-20 µg/kg per minute	Titrate to desired effect
Epinephrine For bradycardia	IV/IO: 0.01 mg/kg (1:10 000) ET: 0.1 mg/kg (1:1000)	Be aware of effective dose of preservatives administered (if preservatives are present in epinephrine preparation) when high doses are used

For asystolic or pulseless arrest	First dose:
	  IV/IO: 0.01 mg/kg
	  (1:10 000)
	  ET: 0.1 mg/kg
	  (1:1000)
	  Doses as high as 0.2 mg/kg may be effective
	Subsequent doses: IV/IO/ET: 0.1 mg/kg
	  (1:1000)
	  Doses as high as 0.2 mg/kg may be effective
		Be aware of effective dose of preservatives administered (if preservatives present in epinephrine preparation) when high doses are used

Epinephrine infusion	Initial at 0.1 µg/kg per minute Higher infusion dose used if asystole present	Titrate to desired effect (0.1-1 µg/kg per minute)
Lidocaine	1 mg/kg per dose	
Lidocaine infusion	20-50 µg/kg per minute	
Sodium bicarbonate	1 mEq/kg per dose or 0.3 × kg × base deficit	Infuse slowly and only if ventilation is adequate

*IV indicates intravenous route; IO, intraosseous route; and ET, endotracheal route.

Table H-3 Preparation of Infusions

Drug	Preparation*	Dose
Epinephrine	0.6 × body weight (kg) equals milligrams added to diluent† to make 100 ml	Then 1 ml/h delivers 0.1 µg/kg/minute; titrate to effect
Dopamine, dobutamine	6 × body weight (kg) equals milligrams added to diluent to make 100 ml	Then 1 ml/h delivers 1 µg/kg/minute; titrate to effect
Lidocaine	120 mg of 40 mg/ml solution added to 97 ml of 5% dextrose in water, yielding 1200 µg/ml solution	Then 1 ml/kg/hour delivers 20 µg/kg/minute

*Standard concentration may be used to provide more dilute or more concentrated drug solution, but then individual dose must be calculated for each patient and each infusion rate:

$$\text{Infusion Rate (ml/h)} = \frac{\text{Weight (kg)} \times \text{Dose (µg/kg/min)} \times 60 \text{ min/h}}{\text{Concentration (µg/mL)}}$$

†Diluent may be 5% dextrose in water, 5% dextrose in half-normal saline, normal saline, or Ringer's lactate.

Figure H-1   Universal Algorithm for Adult Emergency Cardiac Care (ECC)

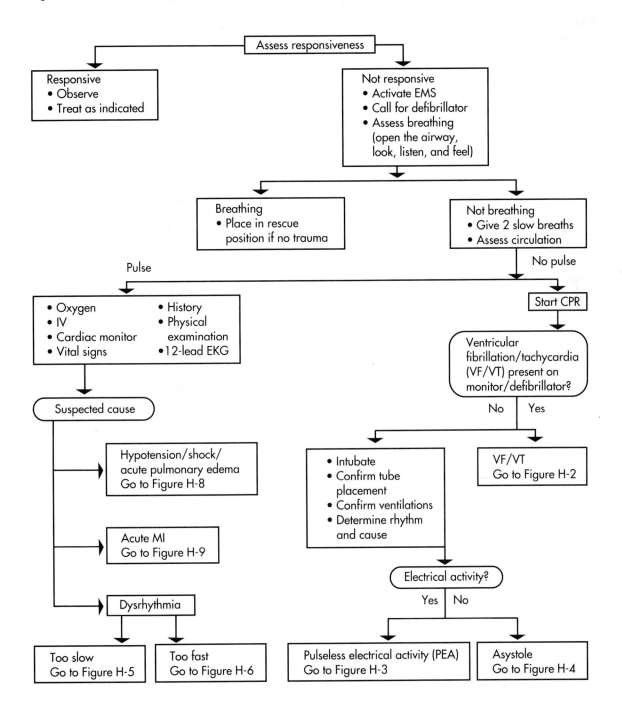

Figure H-2 Algorithm for ventricular fibrillation and pulseless ventricular tachycardia (VF/VT)

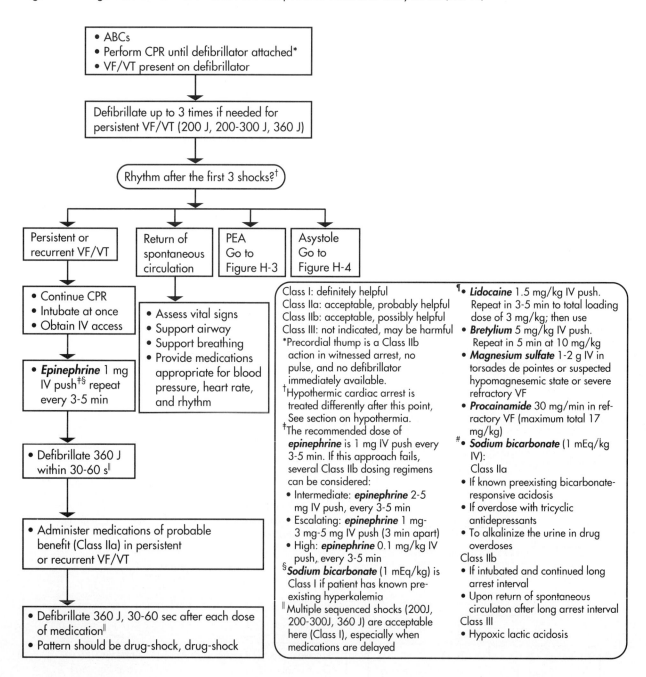

Figure H-3 Algorithm for pulseless electrical activity (PEA) (electromechanical dissociation [EMD])

PEA includes
- Electromechanical dissociation (EMD)
- Pseudo-EMD
- Idioventricular rhythms
- Ventricular escape rhythms
- Bradyasystolic rhythms
- Postdefibrillation idioventricular rhythms

- Continue CPR
- Intubate at once
- Obtain IV access
- Assess blood flow using Doppler ultrasound

⬇

Consider possible causes
(Parentheses=possible therapies and treatments)
- Hypovolemia (volume infusion)
- Hypoxia (ventilation)
- Cardiac tamponade (pericardiocentesis)
- Tension pneumothorax (needle decompression)
- Hypothermia (see hypothermia algorithm, Section IV)
- Massive pulmonary embolism (surgery, **thrombolytics**)
- Drug overdoses such as tricyclics, digitalis, ß-blockers, calcium channel blockers
- Hyperkalemia*
- Acidosis[†]
- Massive acute myocardial infarction
(go to Figure H-9)

⬇

- **Epinephrine** 1 mg IV push,*[†] repeat every 3-5 min

⬇

- If absolute bradycardia (<60 beats/min) or relative bradycardia, give **atropine** 1 mg IV
- Repeat every 3-5 min up to a total of 0.04 mg/kg[§]

Class I: definitely helpful
Class IIa: acceptable, probably helpful
Class IIb: acceptable, possibly helpful
Class III: not indicated, may be harmful
***Sodium bicarbonate** 1 mEq/kg is Class I if patient has known preexisting hyperkalemia.
[†]**Sodium bicarbonate** 1 mEq/kg:
Class IIa
- If known preexisting bicarbonate-responsive acidosis
- If overdose with tricyclic antidepressants
- To alkalinize the urine in drug overdoses
Class IIb
- If intubated and long arrest interval
- Upon return of spontaneous circulation after long arrest interval
Class III
- Hypoxic lactic acidosis
[†]The recommended dose of **epinephrine** is 1 mg IV push every 3-5 min.
If this approach fails, several Class IIb dosing regimens can be considered.
- Intermediate: **epinephrine** 2-5 mg IV push, every 3-5 min
- Escalating: **epinephrine** 1 mg-3 mg-5 mg IV push (3 min apart)
- High: **epinephrine** 0.1 mg/kg IV push, every 3-5 min
[§]Shorter **atropine** dosing intervals are possibly helpful in cardiac arrest (Class IIb).

Figure H-4 Asystole treatment algorithm

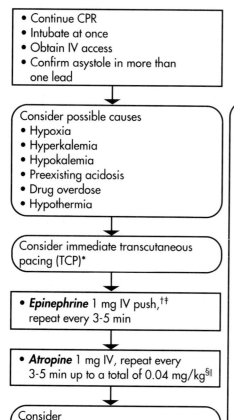

- Continue CPR
- Intubate at once
- Obtain IV access
- Confirm asystole in more than one lead

↓

Consider possible causes
- Hypoxia
- Hyperkalemia
- Hypokalemia
- Preexisting acidosis
- Drug overdose
- Hypothermia

↓

Consider immediate transcutaneous pacing (TCP)*

↓

- **Epinephrine** 1 mg IV push,†‡ repeat every 3-5 min

↓

- **Atropine** 1 mg IV, repeat every 3-5 min up to a total of 0.04 mg/kg§‖

↓

Consider
- Termination of efforts¶

Class I: definitely helpful
Class IIa: acceptable, probably helpful
Class IIb: acceptable, possibly helpful
Class III: not indicated, may be harmful
*TCP is a Class IIb intervention. Lack of success may be due to delays in pacing. To be effective TCP must be performed early, simultaneously with drugs. Evidence does not support routine use of TCP for asystole.
†The recommended dose of **epinephrine** is 1 mg IV push every 3-5 min. If this approach fails, several Class IIb dosing regimens can be considered:
- Intermediate: **epinephrine** 2-5 mg IV push, every 3-5 min
- Escalating: **epinephrine** 1 mg-3 mg-5 mg IV push (3 min apart)
- High: **epinephrine** 0.1 mg/kg IV push, every 3-5 min
‡**Sodium bicarbonate** (1 mEq/kg is Class I if patient has known preexisting hyperkalemia.

§Shorter **atropine** dosing intervals are Class IIb in asystolic arrest.
‖**Sodium bicarbonate** 1 mEq/kg:
  Class IIa
- If known preexisting bicarbonate-responsive acidosis
- If overdose with tricyclic antidepressants
- To alkalinize the urine in drug overdoses
  Class IIb
- If intubated and continued long arrest interval
- Upon return of spontaneous circulation after long arrest interval
  Class III
- Hypoxic lactic acidosis
¶If patient remains in asystole or other agonal rhythms after successful intubation and initial medications and no reversible causes are identified, consider termination of resuscitative efforts by a physician. Consider interval since arrest.

Figure H-5 Bradycardia algorithm (with the patient not in cardiac arrest)

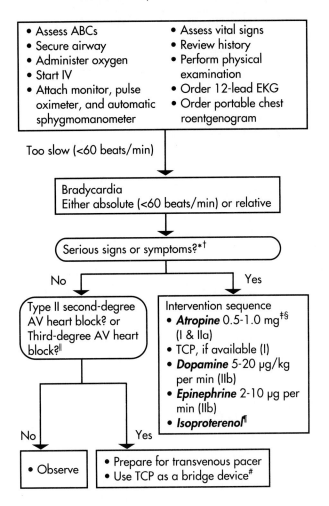

- Assess ABCs
- Secure airway
- Administer oxygen
- Start IV
- Attach monitor, pulse oximeter, and automatic sphygmomanometer
- Assess vital signs
- Review history
- Perform physical examination
- Order 12-lead EKG
- Order portable chest roentgenogram

Too slow (<60 beats/min)

Bradycardia
Either absolute (<60 beats/min) or relative

Serious signs or symptoms?*†

No

Type II second-degree AV heart block? or Third-degree AV heart block?‖

No — • Observe

Yes — • Prepare for transvenous pacer
• Use TCP as a bridge device#

Yes

Intervention sequence
- *Atropine* 0.5-1.0 mg†§ (I & IIa)
- TCP, if available (I)
- *Dopamine* 5-20 µg/kg per min (IIb)
- *Epinephrine* 2-10 µg per min (IIb)
- *Isoproterenol*¶

*Serious signs or symptoms must be related to the slow rate. Clinical manifestations include:
symptoms (chest pain, shortness of breath, decreased level of conciousness) and
signs (low BP, shock, pulmonary congestion, CHF, acute MI).
†Do not delay TCP while awaiting IV access or for *atropine* to take effect if patient is symptomatic.
‡Denervated transplanted hearts will not respond to *atropine.* Go at once to pacing, *catecholamine* infusion, or both.
§*Atropine* should be given in repeat doses in 3-5 min up to total of 0.04 mg/kg. Consider shorter dosing intervals in severe clinical conditions.
It has been suggested that atropine should be used with caution in atrioventricular (AV) block at the His-Purkinje level (type II AV block and new third-degree block with wide QRS complexes) (Class IIb).
‖Never treat third-degree heart block plus ventricular escape beats with *lidocaine.*
¶*Isoproterenol* should be used, if at all, with extreme caution. At low doses it is Class IIb (possibly helpful); at higher doses it is Class III (harmful).
#Verify patient tolerance and mechanical capture. Use analgesia and sedation as needed.

Figure H-6 Tachycardia algorithm

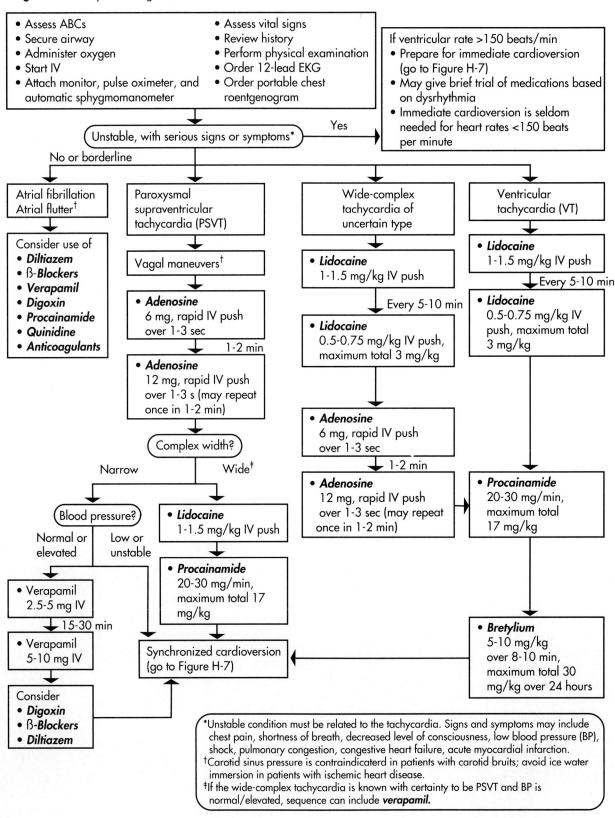

- Assess ABCs
- Secure airway
- Administer oxygen
- Start IV
- Attach monitor, pulse oximeter, and automatic sphygmomanometer

- Assess vital signs
- Review history
- Perform physical examination
- Order 12-lead EKG
- Order portable chest roentgenogram

If ventricular rate >150 beats/min
- Prepare for immediate cardioversion (go to Figure H-7)
- May give brief trial of medications based on dysrhythmia
- Immediate cardioversion is seldom needed for heart rates <150 beats per minute

Unstable, with serious signs or symptoms*   Yes

No or borderline

Atrial fibrillation Atrial flutter†

Consider use of
- *Diltiazem*
- *ß-Blockers*
- *Verapamil*
- *Digoxin*
- *Procainamide*
- *Quinidine*
- *Anticoagulants*

Paroxysmal supraventricular tachycardia (PSVT)

Vagal maneuvers†

- *Adenosine* 6 mg, rapid IV push over 1-3 sec
                    1-2 min
- *Adenosine* 12 mg, rapid IV push over 1-3 s (may repeat once in 1-2 min)

Complex width?

Narrow   Wide†

Blood pressure?   - *Lidocaine* 1-1.5 mg/kg IV push

Normal or elevated   Low or unstable

- Verapamil 2.5-5 mg IV
        15-30 min
- Verapamil 5-10 mg IV

Consider
- *Digoxin*
- *ß-Blockers*
- *Diltiazem*

- *Procainamide* 20-30 mg/min, maximum total 17 mg/kg

Synchronized cardioversion (go to Figure H-7)

Wide-complex tachycardia of uncertain type

- *Lidocaine* 1-1.5 mg/kg IV push
        Every 5-10 min
- *Lidocaine* 0.5-0.75 mg/kg IV push, maximum total 3 mg/kg
- *Adenosine* 6 mg, rapid IV push over 1-3 sec
        1-2 min
- *Adenosine* 12 mg, rapid IV push over 1-3 sec (may repeat once in 1-2 min)

Ventricular tachycardia (VT)

- *Lidocaine* 1-1.5 mg/kg IV push
        Every 5-10 min
- *Lidocaine* 0.5-0.75 mg/kg IV push, maximum total 3 mg/kg
- *Procainamide* 20-30 mg/min, maximum total 17 mg/kg
- *Bretylium* 5-10 mg/kg over 8-10 min, maximum total 30 mg/kg over 24 hours

*Unstable condition must be related to the tachycardia. Signs and symptoms may include chest pain, shortness of breath, decreased level of consciousness, low blood pressure (BP), shock, pulmonary congestion, congestive heart failure, acute myocardial infarction.
†Carotid sinus pressure is contraindicaterd in patients with carotid bruits; avoid ice water immersion in patients with ischemic heart disease.
‡If the wide-complex tachycardia is known with certainty to be PSVT and BP is normal/elevated, sequence can include *verapamil.*

Figure H-7 Electrical cardioversion algorithm (with the patient not in cardiac arrest)

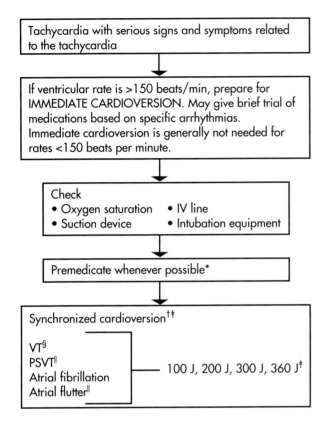

Tachycardia with serious signs and symptoms related to the tachycardia

If ventricular rate is >150 beats/min, prepare for IMMEDIATE CARDIOVERSION. May give brief trial of medications based on specific arrhythmias. Immediate cardioversion is generally not needed for rates <150 beats per minute.

Check
- Oxygen saturation
- Suction device
- IV line
- Intubation equipment

Premedicate whenever possible*

Synchronized cardioversion†‡

VT§
PSVT‖
Atrial fibrillation
Atrial flutter‖

— 100 J, 200 J, 300 J, 360 J†

*Effective regimens have included a sedative (eg, *diazepam, midazolam, barbiturates, etomidate, ketamine, methohexital*) with or without an analgesic agent (eg, *fentanyl, morphine, meperidine*). Many experts recommend anesthesia if service is readily available.
†Note possible need to resynchronize after each cardioversion.
‡If delays in synchronization occur and clinical conditions are critical, go to immediate unsynchronized shocks.
§Treat polymorphic VT (irregular form and rate) like VF: 200 J, 200-300 J, 360 J.
‖ PSVT and atrial flutter often respond to lower energy levels (start with 50 J).

Figure H-8 Algorithm for hypotension, shock, and acute pulmonary edema

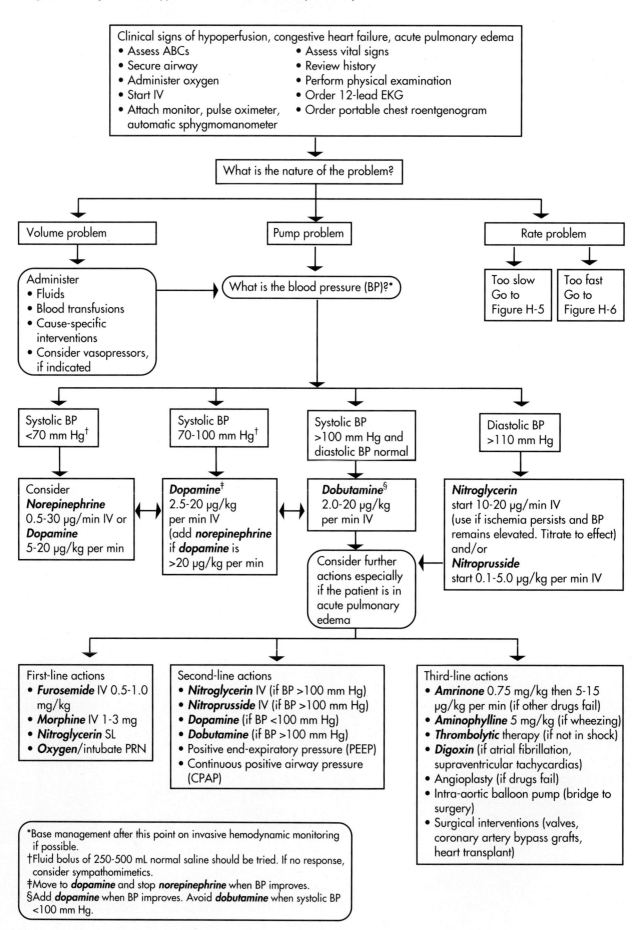

Clinical signs of hypoperfusion, congestive heart failure, acute pulmonary edema
- Assess ABCs
- Secure airway
- Administer oxygen
- Start IV
- Attach monitor, pulse oximeter, automatic sphygmomanometer
- Assess vital signs
- Review history
- Perform physical examination
- Order 12-lead EKG
- Order portable chest roentgenogram

What is the nature of the problem?

Volume problem | Pump problem | Rate problem

Administer
- Fluids
- Blood transfusions
- Cause-specific interventions
- Consider vasopressors, if indicated

What is the blood pressure (BP)?*

Too slow
Go to
Figure H-5

Too fast
Go to
Figure H-6

Systolic BP <70 mm Hg†

Systolic BP 70-100 mm Hg†

Systolic BP >100 mm Hg and diastolic BP normal

Diastolic BP >110 mm Hg

Consider
Norepinephrine 0.5-30 µg/min IV or *Dopamine* 5-20 µg/kg per min

Dopamine‡ 2.5-20 µg/kg per min IV (add *norepinephrine* if *dopamine* is >20 µg/kg per min)

Dobutamine§ 2.0-20 µg/kg per min IV

Nitroglycerin start 10-20 µg/min IV (use if ischemia persists and BP remains elevated. Titrate to effect) and/or *Nitroprusside* start 0.1-5.0 µg/kg per min IV

Consider further actions especially if the patient is in acute pulmonary edema

First-line actions
- *Furosemide* IV 0.5-1.0 mg/kg
- *Morphine* IV 1-3 mg
- *Nitroglycerin* SL
- *Oxygen*/intubate PRN

Second-line actions
- *Nitroglycerin* IV (if BP >100 mm Hg)
- *Nitroprusside* IV (if BP >100 mm Hg)
- *Dopamine* (if BP <100 mm Hg)
- *Dobutamine* (if BP >100 mm Hg)
- Positive end-expiratory pressure (PEEP)
- Continuous positive airway pressure (CPAP)

Third-line actions
- *Amrinone* 0.75 mg/kg then 5-15 µg/kg per min (if other drugs fail)
- *Aminophylline* 5 mg/kg (if wheezing)
- *Thrombolytic* therapy (if not in shock)
- *Digoxin* (if atrial fibrillation, supraventricular tachycardias)
- Angioplasty (if drugs fail)
- Intra-aortic balloon pump (bridge to surgery)
- Surgical interventions (valves, coronary artery bypass grafts, heart transplant)

*Base management after this point on invasive hemodynamic monitoring if possible.
†Fluid bolus of 250-500 mL normal saline should be tried. If no response, consider sympathomimetics.
‡Move to *dopamine* and stop *norepinephrine* when BP improves.
§Add *dopamine* when BP improves. Avoid *dobutamine* when systolic BP <100 mm Hg.

Figure H-9 Acute myocardial infarction (AMI) algorithm. Recommendations for early treatment of patients with chest pain and possible AMI

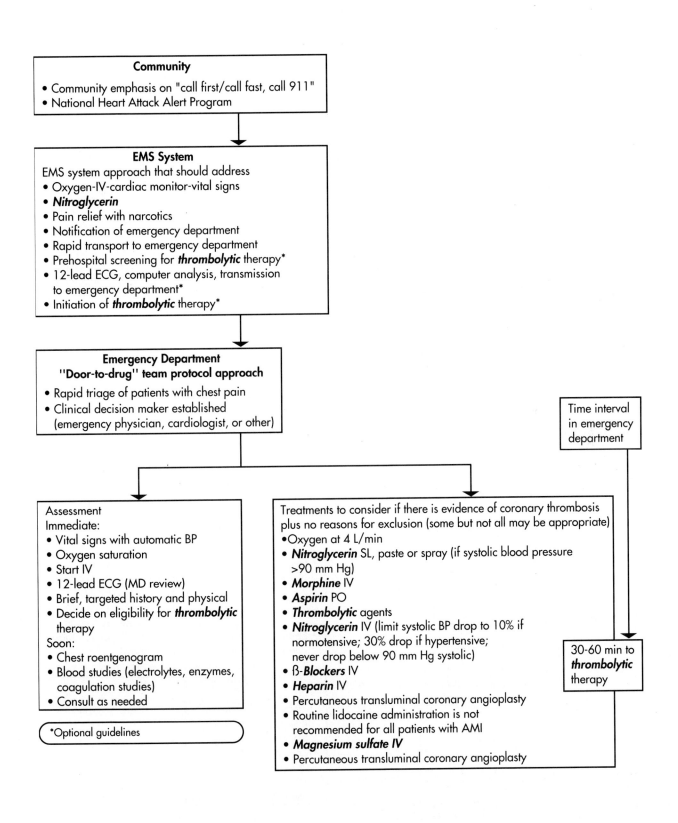

Figure H-10 Pediatric bradycardia decision tree

Figure H-11 Pediatric asystole and pulseless arrest decision tree

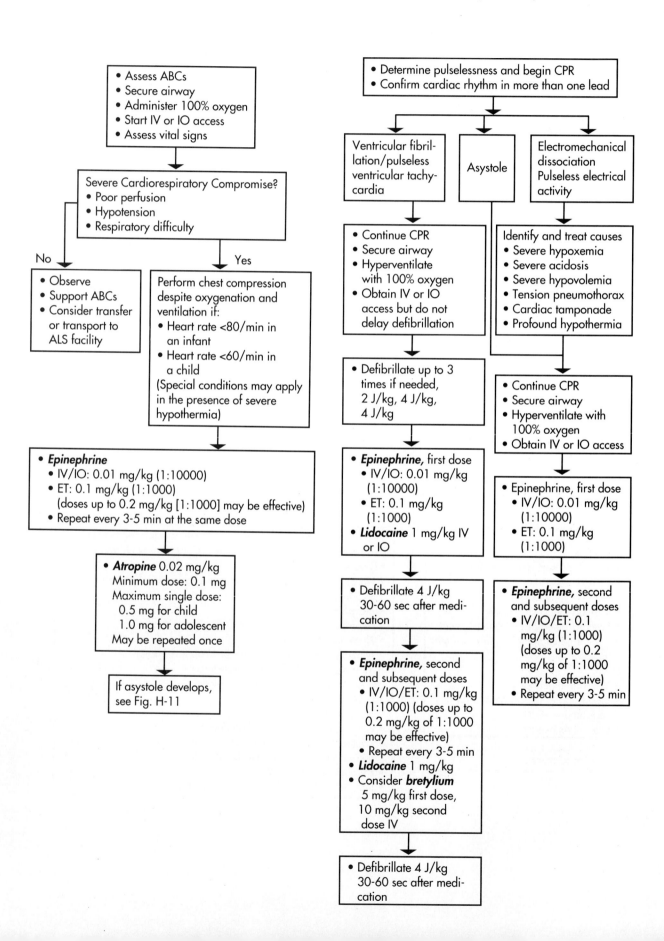

Index

OTHER MOSBY PRODUCTS
OF INTEREST

BOOK CODE	AUTHOR/TITLE	PUBDATE
21764	ACLS: Video Series	12/91
21766	ACLS: Airway Management	12/91
21771	ACLS: Arrhythmia Interpretation	12/91
21772	ACLS: Conversion Techniques	12/91
21770	ACLS: ECG Recognition	12/91
21767	ACLS: IV Procedures	12/91
21765	ACLS: Mega Code	12/91
21768	ACLS: Pharmacology, Part I	12/91
21769	ACLS: Pharmacology, Part II	12/91
07067	American Red Cross CPR for the Professional Rescuer Text	3/93
21231	American Red Cross Emergency Response Text	3/93
21135	American Red Cross First Aid: Responding to Emergencies	3/91
07405	American Safety Video Publishers: Learning ECGs Video Series	10/93
07172	American Safety Video Publishers: PALS Plus: Pediatric Advanced Life Support	12/92
07296	American Safety Video Publishers: PALS Plus: Pediatric Emergencies	12/92
07257	American Safety Video Publishers: Pass ACLS	12/92
00258	Atwood: Introduction to Cardiac Dysrhythmias	3/90
00383	Auerbach-Geehr: Management of Wilderness and Environmental Emergencies, 2/e	12/88
00385	Auf der Heide: Disaster Response	6/89
01185	Bosker: The 60-Second EMT	11/87
01808	Bosker: Geriatric Emergency Medicine	7/90
01330	Bronstein: Emergency Care for Hazardous Materials Exposure	5/88
01458	doCarmo: Basic EMT Skills and Equipment	8/88
01473	Emergidose Slideguides: Pocket Adult/Pediatric Emergency Drugs Guide, 5/e	7/91
01478	Emergidose Slideguides: Binder Adult/Pediatric Emergency Drugs Guide, 5/e	7/91
01472	Emergidose Slideguides: Pocket Pediatric/Neonatal Emergency Drugs Guide, 2/e	8/91
01471	Emergidose Slideguides: Binder Pediatric/Neonatal Emergency Drugs, 2/e	7/91
01969	Gonsoulin: Prehospital Drug Therapy	9/93
01932	Gosselin-Smith: Mosby's First Responder Workbook, 2/e	10/88
	Preparation and a Comprehensive Review, 2/e	8/87
01979	Grauer: ACLS Volume 1, Volume 2, and Pocket Reference	3/93